Blood Pressure Solution

(Two Book Box Set)

Mark Evans

The following Book is reproduced below with the goal of providing information that is as accurate and as reliable as possible. Regardless, purchasing this Book can be seen as consent to the fact that both the publisher and the author of this book are in no way experts on the topics discussed within, and that any recommendations or suggestions made herein are for entertainment purposes only. Professionals should be consulted as needed before undertaking any of the action endorsed herein.

This declaration is deemed fair and valid by both the American Bar Association and the Committee of Publishers Association and is legally binding throughout the United States.

Furthermore, the transmission, duplication or reproduction of any of the following work, including precise information, will be considered an illegal act, irrespective whether it is done electronically or in print. The legality extends to creating a secondary or tertiary copy of the work or a recorded copy and is only allowed with express written consent of the Publisher. All additional rights are reserved.

The information in the following pages is broadly considered to be a truthful and accurate account of facts, and as such any inattention, use or misuse of the information in question by the reader will render any resulting actions solely under their purview. There are no scenarios in which the publisher or the original author of this work can be in any fashion deemed liable for any hardship or damages that may befall them after undertaking information described herein.

Additionally, the information found on the following pages is intended for informational purposes only and should thus be considered, universal. As befitting its nature, the information presented is without assurance regarding its continued validity or interim quality. Trademarks that mentioned are done without written consent and can in no way be considered an endorsement from the trademark holder.

Table of Contents

BLOOD PRESSURE SOLUTION

Introduction...8

Chapter 1: Understanding High Blood Pressure 9

   Reading Blood Pressure...10

   Types of High Blood Pressure 11

Chapter 2: The Silent Killer..13

   When to Start Checking..13

   Risk Factors for Hypertension 14

   Complications of High Blood Pressure 16

Chapter 3: Diet and Blood Pressure 18

   The Importance Of Staying Away From High Sodium Food 18

   What to Eat 19

   Do's and Don'ts In Cooking...25

   What to Avoid 27

Chapter 4: Exercise for Hypertension 29

   Get Doctor's Approval First...29

   Cardio, Strength Training, and Stretching 29

   The Right Way to Exercise 31

Chapter 5: Weight Loss and Hypertension...................................32

Chapter 6: Supplements and Medications that Help.....................34

Chapter 7: Stress and High Blood Pressure..................................38

Chapter 8: Sample Recipes for Lower Blood Pressure..................42

   Breakfast 42

   Lunch...44

   Dinner 49

   Food Substitution 58

Chapter 9: Living With High Blood Pressure - Eating Out..............60

Conclusion 64

BLOOD PRESSURE SOLUTION

Introduction 66
The Dangers of a Rising Blood Pressure 67
   Complications of Hypertension 67
   Symptoms of High Blood Pressure 73
   Things that Raise your Blood Pressure......................... 73
Breakfast Recipes 76
   During the course of the night Chia Oatmeal................ 76
   Sarah's Easy Homemade Applesauce 76
   Egg Scramble 78
   Beer Batter Crepes.. 80
   Sausage Egg Muffins 82
   Ultimate Irresistible Granola...................................... 83
   Banana Bran Muffins 85
   Wake Up Smoothie.. 87
   Cinnamon Bake Donuts 88
   French Toast 90
   Breakfast Power Balls.. 91
   Frozen Fruit Cups... 92
   Vanilla Bean Coconut Yogurt Smoothie 92
   Almond-Honey Power Bar 94
   Orange Resolution Smoothie 96
   Creamy Kale and Eggs... 97
Lunch Recipes 98
   Grilled Sweet Potato and Scallion Salad....................... 98
   Israeli Couscous Tabouli 100
   Frittata with Asparagus, Tomato, and Fontina 101
   Un-fried Chicken 102
   Chicken and Rice Paprikash Casserole......................... 104
   Tropical Chicken Patties 106
   Healthy Summer Pasta Salad....................................... 108
   Chicken Peanut Stir-Fry.. 109
   Kale and Turkey Rice Bowl 111
   Escarole with Pancetta 113
Snack and Side Recipes.. 114
   Roasted Sweet Potatoes with Honey and Cinnamon 114

Garlic Mashed Cauliflower 115
Strawberry Oatmeal Bars 116
Fresh Corn Salad... 117
Kale Chips 118
Pomegranate Quinoa Pilaf.. 119
Healthy Cauliflower Rice 121
Vanilla Almonds.. 122
Watermelon and Cucumber Smoothie................................... 123
Slow Cooker Spiced Nuts.. 124
Spicy Summer Squash with Herbs 125
Pumpkin-Parmesan Biscuits 126
Potatoes with Chili Butter 128
Tomato Gratin.. 129
Eggplant Caponata.. 130
Italian Lentil Salad... 131
Dinner Recipes 133
Oven Baked Salmon.. 133
Pork Tenderloin with Seasoned Rub.....................................135
Mushroom Stuffer Pork Tenderloin 136
Four-Step Lemon-Onion Chicken 138
Dry Rubbed London Broil 140
Herbed Tuna Steaks...141
Steamed Shrimp Dumplings 142
Braised Chicken with Mushrooms 144
Coffee Rubbed Steak with Peppers and Onions 146
Dessert Recipes.. 148
Angel Food Cake 148
Cocoa Brownies.. 150
Lemon Ricotta Cookies with Lemon Glaze 151
Espresso Chip Meringues 153
Healthy No-Bake Chocolate Peanut Butter Bars 154
Greek Yogurt Cheesecake 156
Apple and Berry Brown Betty... 158
Chewy Gluten Free Chocolate Chip Cookies......................... 160
Jam-and-Oat Squares... 162
Conclusion 163
Thank you! 164

BLOOD PRESSURE SOLUTION

THE ULTIMATE GUIDE TO NATURALLY LOWERING HIGH BLOOD PRESSURE AND REDUCING HYPERTENSION

Introduction

Are you suffering from high blood pressure or simply want to guard against this particular health issue? While high blood pressure is one of the most common problems experienced by Americans today, you'll be glad to know that it's completely treatable. The condition is well-researched and thus, the medical community offers a wide range of treatments for hypertension starting from the natural to the drugs.

In this book, you should be able to find out exactly what to do in order to better handle high blood pressure. A condition that comes and goes on practically a daily basis, hypertension is something that must be monitored often in order to ensure that it doesn't lead to complications overtime.

Here's what you should know about high blood pressure!

Chapter 1: Understanding High Blood Pressure

High blood pressure or hypertension is one of the most prevalent health issues in the world today. In the United States, roughly 32 percent of Americans are diagnosed with the condition.

What Is It?

High blood pressure is characterized by an excessive pressure of the blood hitting the organs overtime, therefore causing damage. Think about water running out of your shower which hits the body, causing a gentle 'massage' that feels good after a long hard day. High blood pressure or hypertension creates a 'pressure' that's much stronger than that, only this time, it hits the artery walls of your heart. Although you cannot feel it, this constant pummeling of blood causes damage to the arteries. This is why people diagnosed with high blood pressure have a higher risk of heart disease and stroke.

Compared to Low Blood Pressure

While hypertension is the high pressure of the blood, hypotension is when blood pressure is too low in the body. Both are considered to be health issues although study shows that there are more people who have hypertension. In hypotension, the blood pressure is too low that it doesn't pump up enough blood to all the vital organs. This means that the organs are deprived of much needed oxygen, vitamins, and minerals – causing limitations in how you function.

It's important to understand the significance of the two because people who have hypertension tend to overmedicate, causing them to have a reading of low blood pressure. The goal of this book is to help you keep your blood pressure stays within the normal range.

In any case, the ideal blood pressure should be more than 90/60mmHg but less than 120/80mmHg. This is true for ALL persons regardless of their age and gender. Anything lower than said amount would be considered hypotension.

Pre-hypertension is anything higher than 120/80mmHg but lower than 140/90mmHg. While a reading within this range is still considered normal, you are often advised to take it easy because it's one step away from full blown high blood pressure. Hence, any reading beyond 140/90mmHg will be considered as hypertension.

Reading Blood Pressure

Since hypertension is primarily asymptomatic, meaning it doesn't pose any obvious symptoms, it becomes important for high-risk individuals to check their blood pressure on a routine basis. There are several known ways to check blood pressure today and it pays to have one right at home instead of going to a clinic to have your BP checked.

The first one is a manual method of checking which involve the use of a stethoscope, a pump, a cuff, and a pressure reader. This is an old school reader that is considered to be more accurate than most. Unfortunately, it requires a bit of practice to use and can be tough to use on your own.

Most people therefore opt for a digital type of blood pressure reader. While not 100% accurate, a digital BP reader has minimal margin of error, especially when maintained regularly.

It is also wonderfully convenient in that you can strap it on your wrist and let the BP reader do its job.

Of the two however, it is the manual method that is best used and consistently practiced in hospitals in the interest of accuracy.

Types of High Blood Pressure

It must be noted that while high blood pressure can be a health problem by itself, there are instances when it's actually a symptom of something else. There are two types of high blood pressure right now:

Primary Hypertension

Primary Hypertension is perhaps the most common one in which there's really no specific reason for the condition. This is the type that develops over the years as a person enters his 30s or 40s.

Secondary Hypertension

This type is triggered by an underlying condition - hence, it's actually a symptom of something else. Secondary hypertension can be an indication of any of the following:

- Kidney problems
- Thyroid problems
- Obstructive sleep apnea
- Congenital defect in blood vessels
- Alcohol abuse
- Use of illegally drugs
- Adrenal gland tumors

- Certain medications

Resistant Hypertension

Resistant Hypertension is a situation whereby an individual has taken at least 3 types of medication for high blood pressure – one of which is a diuretic – without any positive results. This kind of hypertension is tough to treat and usually means that there are secondary causes that medicine alone will not be able to handle. Once a patient is diagnosed with Resistant Hypertension, doctors will look further into the condition and check out whether any of the following situations are present:

- Problems with the hormone that helps control blood pressure
- Obstructive sleep apnea
- Obesity
- High intake of alcohol or use of cigarette
- Renal artery stenosis which is a condition wherein there is an accumulation of plaque lining the blood vessels

Chapter 2: The Silent Killer

Hypertension is known as the Silent Killer because it is mainly asymptomatic. This means that there are no obvious symptoms and people who have hypertension rarely show of any symptoms even if they're reaching dangerous levels.

For some people, hypertension produces certain symptoms such as headache, nosebleed, pain on the back of the neck, and shortness of breath. Unfortunately, these symptoms aren't specific and thus would be hard to diagnose. This is why instead of waiting for signs, high-risk people are simply told to routinely check their BP to make sure that they're still within the normal range. Blood pressure checks are also part of the typical doctor's appointment.

When to Start Checking

Once a person hits 18 years of age, BP checks should be done at least once every two years. Those who are in their 40s should have the check once every year. If you're genetically predisposed to high blood pressure or fall within the 'high risks' individuals, then a BP check must be done once a year, even if you're just in your 20s.

Fortunately, blood pressure checks are done so quickly and so easily that there's no need to adhere to the "yearly" routine. This is especially so since blood pressure can change on a daily, weekly, or even monthly basis. Hence, you'll be able to check your BP as often as once a day if you own a digital BP reader.

Individuals who have been diagnosed with high blood pressure are often scheduled for more frequent readings.

Risk Factors for Hypertension

So who are those who are at high risk for hypertension? If you fall within any of the following – chances are you'll need to be checked for hypertension on a routine basis:

- Gender and Age – as people grow older; their risk of hypertension climbs higher. People who are in their 40s are more likely to suffer from the condition. Men tend to develop the condition when they hit 45 years of age. For women, the chances of high blood pressure are more prevalent as they enter 65 years of age.
- Genetics – also note that hypertension tends to run in families. If your parents are diagnosed with high blood pressure, chances are you will too at some point.
- Race – blacks are more likely to suffer from high blood pressure compared to whites.
- Physical Inactivity – heart rates of people who are physically inactive are usually faster, which means that there's more pressure of the blood with the increased pumping force of the heart.
- Being Overweight – physical inactivity also increases the chances of being overweight which in turn increases the likelihood of high blood pressure. More fat means that the heart has to work harder in order to properly distribute the blood all over the body. Hence, it necessitates a faster pumping action that increases blood pressure.
- Too Much Salt – studies have shown that a salty diet can increase the risk of high blood pressure. This is mainly due to the fact that more salt means greater water retention, increasing blood pressure.
- Alcohol – alcohol can also increase your risks of high blood pressure although this is only true for heavy drinkers. Individuals who drink many and often will

14

experience hypertension because alcohol causes heart damage. Moderation is the key with men and women advised to drink no more than 1 or 2 glasses of alcohol per day. Note though that this varies depending on the alcohol you're taking. One serving usually means 12 ounces of beer, 1.5 ounces of any 80-proof liquor and 5 ounces of wine.

- Cigarette – use of cigarette immediately raises the blood pressure due to the chemicals contained in cigarette. It can also cause damage to the arteries, narrowing the lining so that blood is pushed out harder for a higher blood pressure. Note that even secondhand smoke can do this.

- Too Little Vitamin D or Potassium – insufficient amounts of potassium and vitamin D has also been found to increase the risks of high blood pressure. Potassium works primarily to balance sodium levels in the body, which means that too little of this will lead to a rise in your sodium levels. Vitamin D on the other hand is used by the body in producing an enzyme that helps regulate blood pressure.

- Stress – perhaps one of the biggest culprit when it comes to hypertension, it has been shown that people with high-stress jobs tend to suffer more often from high blood pressure.

- Certain Conditions – some health problems can also trigger high blood pressure or have the condition as a symptom. Examples include kidney disease, diabetes and sleep apnea. Pregnant women may also suffer from the said condition.

Complications of High Blood Pressure

When left undetected and untreated, high blood pressure can lead to the following complications:

- Stroke or Heart Attack – perhaps the most common complication, hypertension leads to the thickening or the hardening of the arteries. When this happens, it becomes doubly hard for the heart to push blood through the vessels. Even worse, the chances of blockage become more prevalent, leading to a stroke or a heart attack.

- Heart Failure – as opposed to a heart attack, a heart failure is characterized by the inability of the heart to function properly. Again, this may stem from the fact that the arteries have thickened, making it incredibly difficult from the heart to pump and distribute blood.

- Vision Loss – if blood pressure is consistently high, it can eventually cause damage to the vessels. The blood vessels bringing nutrients to the eye is perhaps one of the more vulnerable ones in the body, which means that it can be easily damaged. When this happens, individuals may experience vision loss.

- Metabolic Issues – the consistent high pressure of the blood can also trigger certain conditions relating to a person's metabolism. For example, it can lead to high cholesterol levels, heart disease, and diabetes. More often than not, the complication of high cholesterol and diabetes go hand in hand with high blood pressure.

- Aneurysm – a ruptured aneurysm can be life threatening and unfortunately, it's typically hard to figure out that one exists. This condition is characterized by the weakening and the bulging of the blood vessels which can pop and result to blood loss.

- Psychological Issues – high blood pressure is also linked

with mental and psychological issues such as difficulty understanding or retaining information.

Since blood goes everywhere, the complications arising out of high blood pressure are numerous.

Chapter 3: Diet and Blood Pressure

Generally, people will suffer from high blood pressure several times during their lifetime. Hypertension is a condition that comes and goes – making it necessary to monitor the same on a routine basis. While your blood pressure may be normal today, it may not be normal tomorrow – which is why a continuing treatment is often important.

Efforts to lower blood pressure is therefore a day to day basis, making it crucial to watch what you eat EVERYDAY.

The good news is that like most conditions, a healthy and balanced diet SHOULD help lower the risks of hypertension. There are certain food items that increase the risk and there are some that have been proven to help you better than others can.

The Importance Of Staying Away From High Sodium Food

Sodium is one of the most common culprits of hypertension. High sodium food items are therefore best avoided if you want to maintain normal blood pressure levels. The problem is that most people see sodium and think 'salt'.

The misconception is that if food is not salty, it's not high in sodium – which is completely false. Even the typical hamburger contains 497mg of sodium and it's not salty at all. This is because sodium is often used to preserve food – which means that ALL PROCESSED food items contain sodium. This includes canned goods, fruit preserves, meat, and more.

In case you're wondering – the absolute limit for daily sodium intake is set at 2300mg per day. For people who want to lower or maintain their blood pressure however, it should NOT BE MORE THAN 1500mg per day. Unfortunately, most people today eat more than 2300mg through processed food items.

Some delicacies however are more dangerous than others. Later in the book, we will talk more about what NOT to eat.

What to Eat

So what should you eat now if you can't consume processed food? Following are some items that are known for their positive effect on blood pressure:

Banana

Although not exactly a cure-all for diseases, banana is undoubtedly one of the healthiest fruits available today. A single banana contains 12 percent of the potassium you'll need for the day, 8 percent of the magnesium and 1 percent of the calcium. There are also news today saying that bananas, especially the ones with black spotting on the skin, can help prevent cancer. This is why it's a good idea to chop up your overripe bananas and store them in the freezer for a satisfying shake! Aside from its potassium content, banana is also known for lowering stress levels in the body.

Avocado

Currently viewed as a power food, avocado isn't as nutritious as the media claims it to be. However, that doesn't mean that you should skip eating this fruit! When given the opportunity, make sure to grab some avocado for your kitchen because this contains 10% of your daily potassium requirements.

White Beans

The great thing about white beans is that you can add them to practically all types of recipes, introducing a new twist to your favorite food items. A cup of white beans contains 13% of the calcium you need and 24% of the potassium you need on a daily basis. Serve them with some shrimp and you should be able to keep your sodium and calorie levels low.

Papaya

Very few people take a good look at papaya for lowering high blood pressure. This tropical fruit will surprise you however due to its high vitamin C content – not to mention its delicious taste. While papaya is often eaten ripe or when it is already very orange in coloring, there are those who prefer this fruit while they are still ripening. In the green-orange stage, you'll find that the crunchy flesh can be pleasurable to eat. Either way however, papaya is a good source of vitamins and minerals making it an excellent snack.

Cantaloupe

The bad news is that when it comes to potassium content, nothing really beats banana. This is why you'll need to consume as much as half a cantaloupe in order to get the same amount of potassium in a banana. Still, that's not bad considering the additional minerals and vitamins you'll be getting. Cantaloupe is also known for its antioxidant content which helps the body with the healing process.

Broccoli and Kale

These two are lumped together because they're both green and leafy. They're also highly nutritious with broccoli containing 14% of your daily potassium needs while kale adds 9% more. Together, they can lower your blood pressure, increase your fiber intake, and essentially boost your body's immune system. Broccoli has the added benefit of containing cancer-fighting minerals. Although they not exactly great taste, you'll find that the right recipe will make these greens more gorgeous for the taste buds. You can also try adding them in a daily green shake for better results.

Kiwi

Something you can purchase the whole year round, Kiwis have more vitamin C in them compared to an orange of the same size. There's also the fact that they taste heavenly and are much easier to split open if you know the life hack for it. This contains roughly 9% of the potassium you need on a daily basis.

Tomatoes

Tomatoes offer a multitude of benefits, one of which is lowering high blood pressure. Bear in mind though that just because the product is made from tomato, it's already 'healthy'. For example, canned tomatoes contain so much sodium. The same goes for canned tomato sauce for pizza. Hence, it's usually better to eat tomatoes raw – perhaps toss them in a salad or enjoy the fruit as it is. You can also add it to main dishes and take advantage of the unique taste offered by the product.

Oatmeal

While oatmeal is generally healthy, you have to be careful about what kind of oatmeal you're eating in the first place. Flavored ones aren't really a good idea since they contain more sugar than the regular kind. The solution: try to add your own sweetener to the oatmeal. Honey is always an excellent choice because it is beautifully natural. You can also add fruit like strawberries and berries to make the taste more engaging. It quickly fills the stomach and if you're not a fan of the food, you can limit consumption to just one big bowl for breakfast.

Low Fat Dairy

A study published in the Journal of Human Hypertension shows that consumption of dairy helps reduce the chances of hypertension. It should only be low-fat dairy however since high-fat dairy contains more saturated fat which contributes to hypertension. Moderate consumption is still encouraged.

Dark Chocolate

While chocolate is often seen as 'bad', there are actually instances when it's a good thing. Chocolate – particularly the dark kind – contains flavanols which help regulate blood pressure. It's an excellent preventive for those who have pre-hypertension, essentially lowering the pressure so that it doesn't go beyond the limit. Chocolate also has properties that help a person relax and de-stress, allowing for the blood vessels to expand and therefore slow down the flow of the blood.

Blueberries

Another excellent fruit, blueberries are best eaten fresh instead of something you get from a can. In fact, all berries are excellent for people with hypertension, whether they're the 'black' kind or the 'straw' kind. Remember that while blueberries are great, eating them together with other non-great food would dampen the effect of the fruit. For example, if you're going to eat blueberries together with layers of waffle or pancakes drizzle in maple syrup, then you're doing more bad than good.

Drinking Water

Very few people realize just how effective water is in lowering blood pressure. It's a given that you should drink at least 8 glasses a day – but the timing of when you drink water is equally important. It's often best to drink water before and after eating. Drinking water before taking a bath has also been shown to help lower blood pressure. If you've just exercised and lost a ton of water through sweat, make sure to supplement that with an additional glass for the day!

Fatty Fish

Fatty Fish is a rich source of omega-3 fatty acids which is known for lowering cholesterol levels, regulating blood sugar levels, and lowering high blood pressure. Of course, fatty fish aren't the only source of omega-3 fatty acids although they are the most popular. Olive oil is a popular source as well as flaxseed oil, walnut oil, and soybean oil.

Whole Grains

The American Journal of Clinical Nutrition has published the benefits of whole grains when it comes to blood pressure. The study was directed specifically towards middle-aged people who have a high risk of blood pressure. Three servings of the food per day will be enough to produce significant results.

The DASH Diet

The DASH Diet is currently being used for weight loss purposes, but it's actually developed for people with hypertension. In fact, the name stands for "Dietary Approaches to Stop Hypertension."

While some people prefer to simply 'avoid the bad and eat the good', there are those who function better with a planned regimen designed to lower blood pressure. This is where the DASH Diet comes in, offering you set meal plans, time of meals, recipes, and even lifestyle changes that overall contribute towards lower blood pressure.

The general principles of the DASH Diet are the following:

- The diet focuses on eating food low in sodium, fat, and cholesterol while increasing the consumption of protein and fiber.
- Food consumption is limited to the following categories: fruits, vegetable, whole grains, fish, poultry, nuts, and low fat dairy products.
- At the same time, it prohibits overconsumption of red meat, sugar, and sweets.

There's also a fairly specific approach to how you eat. Ideally, the following routine is followed:

- Calorie consumption is limited to just 2,000 a day or depending on the doctor's recommendation.
- There should be 4 to 5 servings of fruit per day
- There should be 6 to 8 servings of grain per day

- There should be 4 to 5 servings of vegetables per day
- There should be 2 to 3 servings of dairy per day
- There should be less than 6 servings of poultry, fish, or lean meat per day
- There should be 2 to 3 servings of fat and oils per day
- There should be less than 5 servings of sweets per week
- There should be 4 to 5 servings of nuts, legumes, and seeds per week

Do's and Don'ts In Cooking

For the most part, cooking for high blood pressure is more than just choosing the right ingredients. Bananas are great – but if you start combining them with ice cream – then this will defeat the purpose of potassium in your diet. That being said, there are some common dos and don'ts when it comes to cooking for hypertension. As long as you follow them, you should be able to experiment your way through blood pressure friendly recipes.

Later on in this book, we'll show you different recipes you can follow to help lower high blood pressure.

- Do roast meat on a rack, allowing the fat to drip off so that you won't consume it
- Instead of frying, try to broil or grill your meat and vegetables – this should produce excellent tasting food without the scary oil
- Steaming is also another excellent way of cooking food quickly, easily, and healthily
- For people with high blood pressure, having a pressure cooker is tantamount to gold. Practically anything can be cooked this way so try to use this as often as possible
- Stew meat first so that the fat is effectively separated

from the meat. Once you've stewed the meat, you can easily store it in the fridge and simply add to any meal you happen to be cooking. This also helps speed up the cooking process since the meat is practically done

- Avoid prepackaged stuff. If you have no other choice, opt for the low-sodium choices
- It's also a good idea to switch sodium for more healthy food items. Here are some excellent alternatives, depending on what kind of food you're cooking:
    - Basil for fish, lean meats, and sauces
    - Chives are a perfect addition to vegetables
    - If you're cooking something rich like potatoes and meatloaf, rosemary should add a certain bite to the meal
    - Make your spaghetti sauce tangy with some cider vinegar
    - Make your food just a little bit spicy by adding paprika
    - Lemon juice – a common favorite and perfect for practically anything from salads, fish, and vegetables

What to Avoid

The list of what food items to avoid are fairly obvious. Unfortunately, there are some things that are less obvious and can be quite confusing for some people. The general rule is that if it's processed, it's bad – regardless of the actual nature of the food. Of course, not all 'fresh' food items are ideal either. Here are some stuff you need to avoid if you want to lower your blood pressure:

Frozen Fish

Fish is undoubtedly a healthy fare – but what if it's frozen or salted? Fish that's been specifically cured to last longer in the shelves are best left alone if you're trying to lower your blood pressure. The same is true for the canned kind – even if it's a healthy tuna fare. Fortunately, there are currently products that are low in sodium so you might want to check them out.

Chinese Food

They might seem healthy, especially with all the broccoli and fish that's included in the menu – but you might be surprised at how proficient the Chinese are in using salt in their meals. One of the most common dips for Chinese Food is Soy Sauce which is just packed with sodium. Even if you choose to skip the soy sauce however, you can be sure that there's still an amazing amount of salt added into the food so you might as well just skip it completely.

Pizza

Pizza is heavy on sodium – even if you do load it up with pineapple pieces to 'balance' the health benefits. Pepperoni alone is already loaded in salt, much less the tomato sauce and the bread. Note though that we previously mentioned how tomato is good for you – but keep in mind that we're referring to fresh tomatoes. When it comes to packed tomato sauce, the sodium content is just as high as anything else. Add the dairy cheese and you've just consumed your one week of sodium quota in one sitting.

Pastries

You'd think that sweet food items don't have salt – but you might be surprised. Cakes, cookies, muffins, and all other types of pastries contain large amounts of sodium which makes them a danger to both diabetics and those with high blood pressure. You can find low-fat options in the market, but it's hardly worth it with so many other healthier options available. Packed pastries are the worst since they're made to last longer on the shelves, thus containing more preservatives – one of which is salt.

Alcohol

This seems like a no-brainer, but lots of people still forget to exclude alcohol in their diet if they're looking to lower blood pressure. While alcohol can be healthy in small dosage, they're not exactly very helpful when taken on a daily basis. If you can't go through a day without some form of alcohol, stick to just one cup of red wine which has been proven to have health benefits.

Chapter 4: Exercise for Hypertension

Proper exercise also contributes largely to hypertension prevention. The good news is that you DON'T have to exercise extensively in order to lower blood pressure. Just a few minutes each day should be able to help with the problem. Even better, there's no need to make a concentrated effort towards exercise. Some of the most common household chores today offer sufficient workout to get the blood pumping.

Get Doctor's Approval First

Since most people who suffer from hypertension are in their later years, it makes sense to first obtain the doctor's approval. Find out the limits of your exercises, how many minutes you can spend each day and what workouts should be avoided to prevent damage to your person. For example, some people are advised against running since this puts remarkable pressure on the knees. Exercising for more than 30 minutes per day can also prove to be dangerous from some people instead of being helpful.

If your doctor has given you the 'go ahead' without any restrictions, then you can follow the guideline given in this book.

Cardio, Strength Training, and Stretching

Cardiovascular or aerobics exercises are by far the best type of exercise for hypertension. They're also great for losing weight and generally attaining a healthier body. This is generally any exercise that gets your heart pumping a little faster such as jogging, swimming, walking, cleaning the house, Zumba, dancing, and so much more. It is best to complement these workouts with strength training to build stronger muscles together with stretching to limit cramps and pain after a good exercise.

How Often to Exercise

The frequency of your exercises should be limited to just 30 minutes a day, done 5 times a week. You can choose when your rest day would be, depending on how busy you are on that particular day. Bear in mind that the intensity of your activity plays a major role here. For example, brisk walking is the kind of moderate activity that commands 30 minutes of exercise for 5 days a week. An intense workout like jogging however offers the same benefit when done 15 minutes for 5 days a week.

The Right Way to Exercise

- Give yourself a 5 to 10 minute warm up which should include stretching, just to get the blood flow started. This will help prevent injury. Make sure that it's a full-body stretching, involving the legs, arms, and back.
- Figure out how long you're supposed to exercise and the intensity of the workout. A treadmill should be useful at this point because it allows you to set up a precise time and speed for the exercise. Of course, other activities should also work for you.
- A good measure of intensity is your capacity to hold a conversation during exercise. Brisk walking should give you enough breath to talk with someone – but not sing. If you can sing while you're working out, you're not pumping up enough energy into the exercise.
- Once you're done, make sure to do another round of stretching. This helps prevent any pain that you might get from the workout or any cramps that might occur due to the shock.

Chapter 5: Weight Loss and Hypertension

You'll notice that exercise and diet are two of the top natural methods to help prevent high blood pressure and these two things have one goal in mind: to help you lose weight. Of course, that doesn't mean that only overweight people suffer from high blood pressure. Even skinny people can have hypertension and for these people, assuming a healthy lifestyle without having to lose weight is acceptable.

If you're overweight however, it's better to lose several pounds together with assuming a healthier lifestyle. But just how much weight should you lose?

Body Mass Index

Body Mass Index or BMI is quite possibly one of the most popular methods in determining whether you're carrying more mass than you're supposed to. BMI is a widely available tool that you can access online. Taking into account factors like your height, weight, age, and gender – it can tell you whether you're underweight, overweight, or just average for your particular height and weight. A healthy BMI is between 18.5 and 25. A person with a BMI of 30 is deemed moderately obese.

For purposes of lowering your high blood pressure, try to lose as much weight as necessary to bring your BMI within normal level and to maintain that healthy level.

Finding Out Your BMI

There are several websites today that offer easy BMI calculation. Check out this link or go to www.smartbmicalculator.com to find out your own.

Additional Benefits of Weight Loss

Since weight loss is considered to be one of the most common risk factors for various diseases, you'll find that by shedding the pounds, you can also decrease the chances of the following health problems:

- Coronary heart disease
- Hypertension
- Sleep apnea
- Stroke
- Osteoarthritis
- Type 2 diabetes
- Certain types of cancer

Chapter 6: Supplements and Medications that Help

While going natural is often better when controlling high blood pressure, the fact is that there are instances when supplements and medications are prescribed by the doctor to get better results. Depending on your hypertension situation, you might find some of the following medicines given to help manage the problem:

Medications Prescribed by Doctors for Treatment

Thiazide Diuretics

Diuretics essentially make it possible for your body to get rid of sodium and water. Sodium in particular can increase instances of high blood pressure, which is why it's important to flush it out of the system. Being relatively safe, diuretics are the first thing doctors prescribe to their patients, especially since it works for practically everyone.

Beta Blockers

This kind of medication is offered in conjunction with other hypertension medicine. They seem to work better when combined with other drugs. Their primary function is to help the heart beat slower, thereby causing less force.

Angiotensin-Converting Enzyme Inhibitors

Also known as ACE Inhibitors, they prevent the narrowing of the blood vessels by inhibiting the chemicals the cause the narrowing process. They essentially cause the blood vessels to relax. The same is accomplished by *Angiotensin II Receptor Blockers* but this one is often given to those with chronic kidney disease.

Calcium Channel Blockers

This has two effects. The first is to relax the blood vessels so more blood can pass through without the extensive pressure. At the same time, it slows down the heart rate to decrease the push of blood through the blood vessels.

Typically, Calcium Channel Blockers are prescribed to African Americans or older individuals who have higher risk of acquiring hyperextension. One warning though: make sure not to eat or drink grapefruit juice when taking calcium channel blockers since it's been known to interact negatively with the medication.

Renin Inhibitors

This helps slow down the process of renin production. Renin is an enzyme created by the kidneys that can trigger high blood pressure. You can think of renin as a vital ingredient in the body's increased risk of hypertension. By removing this ingredient however, the domino effect doesn't start so there's little chance of hypertension.

Vasodilators

As the name suggests, they help the vessels dilate which in turn promotes blood flow. More specifically, they work on the vessels of the heart.

Alpha Beta Blockers and Alpha Blockers

These two medications help reduce nerve impulse to the blood vessels. They work basically the same way but Alpha Beta has the added benefit of slowing down the heart rate.

Central Acting Agents

They help by blocking signals to the brain causing high blood pressure. It indirectly helps prevent increased heart rate and narrowing of the vessels.

Aldosterone Antagonists

They're perfect for those who have too much sodium in their diet. The medication works by limiting sodium retention, known to be a primary cause of hypertension.

Prescriptions as Preventive

This is a list of medications that doesn't necessitate a doctor's prescription. You can purchase them over the counter and know that they would be able to help control your blood pressure – especially when combined with other healthy lifestyle choices.

Aspirin

Aspirin is often taken when blood pressure is already within the 'normal' or 'pre-hypertension' range. This is a preventive against cardiovascular diseases which may arise due to hypertension.

Omega-3 Fatty Acids

You've probably seen how fatty fish is one of the best foods to help lower high blood pressure. The main content of fatty fish crucial for treating hypertension is omega-3 fatty acids. Absent any fatty fish in the market or perhaps if tuna starts to cost more than your rent – you can always purchase a bottle of omega-3 fatty acids supplement. Widely available thanks to their excellent health benefits, omega-3 fatty acids should provide just a little less than your daily recommended dosage – which is more than what most people are getting today.

Olive Oil

The great thing about olive oil is the fact that you can add it to practically anything. Packed with health benefits, olive oil also works towards better blood pressure levels. It's currently one of the top health foods today with nutritionists encouraging many to swap their animal oil for the healthier olive oil. While you can quickly add this to your diet by simply incorporating the oil in practically any recipe, there are also supplements that contain this vital ingredient. Look for "benolea olive leaf extract" which should contain olive oil in acceptable doses. If you can't find any, just make sure to get supplements with olive oil as one of the ingredients.

Grape Seed

Grape seed extract also contains large amounts of polyphenols that can contribute to overall health. When it comes to high blood pressure, grape seed contributes but promoting the relaxation of the muscle tissues and the blood vessels – therefore making it easier for the blood to pass through with very little force. Again, you can easily find grape seed extracts in the supplement section of stores today.

Chapter 7: Stress and High Blood Pressure

Many people see stress as one of the top reasons that their blood pressure gets elevated sky-high. Although stress is definitely a factor, you should bear in mind that it is not as relevant as you think it is. Diet is still the primary reason for high blood pressure and no matter how 'relaxed' you get, a bad diet will always lead to hypertension.

Short Term Results

Stress triggers the release of certain hormones that causes high blood pressure. The results however are fairly short term – which means that this won't be the same in a few hours or days. By itself however, stress cannot cause high blood pressure – which means that pre-existing conditions must also be present with the stress, essentially 'tipping the scales' towards hypertension.

Of course, this doesn't mean that any concerted effort on your part to 'relax' won't produce any results. If you're feeling stressed and want to diminish the chances of getting high blood pressure, there are ways you can lower the stress and therefore the spike in your blood pressure. Here are some tips that should help handle the problem:

Sleep

Sleep it off and get a good night's rest at the same time. You'll find that sleep has a way of equalizing so many things and leaving you feeling rebooted the next day. Of course, stress itself can trigger insomnia or make your sleeping hours restless – which are why it's a good idea to let loose before sleeping. Go out with friends, watch a good movie, or do a little stretching to prepare yourself for sleep.

Massage

One of the best ways to just let loose every single strain living in your muscles, a full body massage should bring you back to zero when it comes to stress. It can be quite expensive though so try to limit your massages to those times when you're really feeling at the end of your tether. Once every month would be perfect.

Exercise

Definitely one of the best ways to relax – a good exercise promotes the release of certain hormones that help you feel good about yourself. Of course, don't forget the fact that exercise in itself is very healthy and helps with weight loss – which is one of the primary reasons for hypertension. Using this technique to 'relax', you're basically hitting several birds with just one very effective stone.

Luxurious Bath

Of course, if you don't want to spend a single dime in order to relax, you can always fill the bath tub and just luxuriate in the feel of lukewarm water relaxing your muscles. Pump up the relaxation levels by adding some bath salts, lighting lavender candles and perhaps listening to soothing music. This is something you can do at least once a week to give you that 'ready' feels when Monday finally comes crawling back.

Efficient Breathing Techniques

You might be surprised at how much you're doing breathing wrong and how well this can help relieve stress if you do it correctly. In Asia, proper breathing is incorporated in practically all kinds of exercise and martial arts in order to maximize the capacity of the body to do its job. It's also been known to help lower heart rate, promote better thinking, improve circulation, and of course – lower blood pressure. When you are not conscious about your breathing, you tend to have a shallower breathing than what you are suppose to have. Be mindful with your breathings. The easiest and simplest way to start breathing properly is to just take about 3-5 seconds to breath in slowly from your nose, then hold your breath for a few seconds, and take about 5-7 seconds to release out the air as well as the tension in your body. You can increase the number of seconds for each step as you get better.

Chiropractic Medicine

It's also a good idea to undergo chiropractic medicine if you want to release some of the tension from your body. Working for prolonged periods of time can lead to pinched nerves, problems with your posture and pain directed to different body parts. Chiropractic medicine should be able to help align any body parts that out of their proper position, thereby relieving any pressure on the nerves. Without any pain brought on by prolonged sitting or standing – you should find it easier to deal with stress.

Of course, those are just some of the relaxation techniques you can use in order to help relieve stress that contributes to high blood pressure. Keep in mind that managing stress is simply a contributory factor to hypertension. It's crucial that you manage to successfully combine this approach with a healthy diet and sufficient exercise.

Chapter 8: Sample Recipes for Lower Blood Pressure

There are currently lots of recipes and dietary plans created for people with high blood pressure. An entirely distinct diet system called DASH is built specifically to handle hypertension. While all of them offer an overview or a pattern that you should follow, others make it easier by providing specific recipes that you can check out.

Here are some suggestions on how you should approach each meal time if you have high blood pressure.

Breakfast

Scrambled Egg Whites
Containing lots of amino acids, egg whites help lower blood pressure according to a study by the American Chemical Society as of 2013. You can eat it as is or add some vegetables to boost the positive effects of meal. The best choices would be spinach and tomatoes since they're packed with potassium and calcium. You can also add dairy product – specifically low fat cheese – to make the meal tastier without ruining your hypertension diet. Cook in as little oil as possible or use a healthier oil alternative.

Yogurt and Fruits
It's literally never a bad idea to eat fresh fruits and if you combine them with yogurt, then that would be so much better! Even just 8 ounces of fat free yogurt will provide 10 percent of your daily potassium and magnesium consumption. Combine this with a banana and you're ready to start the day healthy.

Fruit Muffins, Whole Grain

Emphasis on the 'whole grain' since white flour muffins is NOT good for blood pressure. According to the American Journal of Clinical Nutrition published in the year 2010, fruit whole-grain muffins contain flavonoids which help reduce signs of hypertension. It would be even better if the 'fruit' part involves bananas or raisins since they contain equal amounts of potassium.

Soy Milk

Soy Milk is also a good way to start breakfast although you'd probably want this together with other solid meals. If you're not fond of soy milk, you can always check out freshly squeezed orange juice or simply low fat milk.

Peanut Butter Toast

On the run? Might as well throw some bread in the toaster and lather it up with peanut butter. Despite how 'unhealthy' this might seem, peanut butter on toast is actually a good day starter for people with hypertension. The peanut butter has to be natural however – not something you can grab through any store and is packed with preservatives. The bread should also be whole wheat to really get the positive effects of the item. Add in a bowl of grapes, strawberries, or a banana – whatever fruit takes your fancy.

Salmon Sandwich

Again, we're talking about whole wheat bread here instead of basic white bread. Grab a pouch of salmon and mix it with reduced fat mayonnaise – just one tablespoon would be perfect. Add some celery, chopped onions, and have a side of any fruit you want for a complete breakfast.

Coffee or Tea

Yes – you can drink coffee or tea in the morning although it's often advised that you don't do so – especially if you love to drench it in sugar. If you're going to take any of these drinks, make sure to add soymilk or nonfat milk to even out the bitter taste. As for tea, you can always add a wedge of lemon – this would be better than sugar.

Lunch

Lunch is a tricky part of meal times because you only get one hour to actually do something about your food. Hence, most people try to opt for takeaways during lunch. Here are some lunch ideas you can try doing for that one hour. We've also listed some perfect 'take away' options that are perfect for the busy individual with high blood pressure.

Veggies in Pressure Cooker

A pressure cooker is quite possibly one of the best things to have in the kitchen. They're quick, they're handy, they don't require oil, and they produce some of the best tasting cooked foods in just a few minutes. Add your choice of seasoning but for the most part, a pressure cooker cooks food in such a way that all the best parts of the taste are locked in with the food. Here's a basic guide on how to cook vegetables with a pressure cooker:

- Whole artichokes – 8 to 11 minutes
- Asparagus – 1 to 2 minutes
- Beets – 20 to 25 minutes
- Cabbage, thickly sliced – 3 to 4 minutes
- Carrots, 1 inch slices – 2 to 4 minutes
- Chestnuts – 7 to 9 minutes

- Cauliflower – 2 to 3 minutes
- Celery, 1 inch slices – 2 to 3 minutes
- Eggplants, thick slices – 2 to 3 minutes
- Kale – 1 to 3 minutes
- Okra – 2 to 3 minutes
- Medium potatoes – 5 to 7 minutes
- Pumpkin – 3 to 4 minutes
- Zucchini, thick slices – 1 to 2 minutes

Raspberry on Grilled Chicken

Taking only 30 minutes to prepare, here's what you need for this treat:

- Cooking spray
- ¼ tsp of cayenne
- 4 boneless and skinless chicken, about ½ inch in thickness
- 1 1/3 cup of fresh raspberries
- 2 tbsp of low sodium honey mustard
- ¾ cup of seedless raspberry spread

Start by spraying the grill rack with the cooking spray and preheating it while you get everything ready. Grab a separate bowl and mix together the following: raspberry spread, cayenne, and honey mustard. Set aside around ¼ of a cup and use the remaining ones to coat the chicken on both sides. Grill the chicken for 10 minutes per side.

Once cooked, take out the chicken breast and proceed to coat it with the raspberry mixture that you initially set aside. Top with fresh raspberries and enjoy!

Quinoa, Salmon, and Blueberries

Quinoa is packed with protein and is an excellent alternative to rice or bread. Here's how you prepare this new food for a meal:

- ¼ cup balsamic vinegar
- 1 cup fresh blueberries
- Salmon
- Quinoa

Quinoa is cooked pretty much like rice. Combine 2 parts of water for 1 part quinoa and microwave the whole thing in a bowl for 4 minutes. You can add some flavorings if you like but make sure it's not salt. Onion flakes are a common favorite.

As for the rest, grab a saucepan and boil the balsamic vinegar combined with the blueberries. Allow them to stay there until the water is reduced to at least half of how you originally started. You can go as thick or as thin as you like with this one. Once done, just pour a little bit of the sauce onto the salmon. You can add more fresh raspberries or blueberries on the side. Eat with your quinoa.

Spiced Root Vegetable Wedges

Potatoes are a common favorite and when cooked properly, they're actually very healthy. This recipe calls for a healthy serving of sweet potatoes combined with the very appetizing carrot and parsnips.

Here's what you'll need:

- 2 carrots, large
- 2 parsnips
- 2 tbsp of canola oil
- ½ tsp of ground cinnamon

- 1.5 pounds peeled sweet potatoes
- 2 tbsp of coriander seeds, lightly crushed
- 1 lime, juiced
- Salt and pepper to taste

Total amount of time to get this done would be 1 hour and 30 minutes – which should probably make this a better dinner than lunch. Either way, here's how you go about it:

- Start by preheating the oven to 425 degrees Fahrenheit
- Cut the carrots and parsnips into sticks. Boil them in a saucepan using just enough water to make sure everything is submerged in it. Once they're boiling, lower the fire and partly cover the pan with a lid. Allow them to cook like this for just 2 minutes
- Cut the potatoes into sticks,
- Pay attention to the lime juice, cinnamon, coriander, and salt and pepper this time by mixing them together.
- Coat the potatoes in the spice mixture and set them aside
- Remove the carrot and the parsnips, draining them of water before coating them too in the spice mixture.
- Put the carrots, parsnips, and potatoes in a roasting pan and bake them in the oven. This should take about 40 minutes. Make sure to turn them at least twice to make sure every portion is brown

As for the dip, you can try adding together sugar, lime zest, mustard, dill, and yogurt. Of course, this is completely optional and it would be best if you don't have any dip at all for hypertension purposes.

Hash Browns

When it comes to high blood pressure, the rule of thumb is to bake instead of fry. Here's an excellent oven baked hash brown recipe:

- ¼ tsp black pepper
- Cooking spray
- 4 cup shredded baking potato
- ¼ cup green onions, thinly sliced
- ¼ cup green pepper, chopped
- 2 tbsp cornstarch
- ¼ tsp onion powder
- ¼ tsp salt

Start by preheating the oven to 475 degrees Fahrenheit. While the oven is getting ready, put the potato in a large bowl and cover it with cold water for 5 minutes. Drain, rinse, and pat it dry completely.

Grab a bowl and combine the bell pepper, onions, and potato together. Mix in the salt, black pepper, onion powder and cornstarch. Make sure that the potato is well mixed into it.

Grab a baking sheet and line it with aluminum foil before spraying some cooking spray generously. Now use a biscuit cutter to shape your hash browns by carefully filling them and then removing the cutter. Try not to pack the hash brown together but just let it sit comfortably onto the baking sheet. Don't put in more than ½ cup of potato mixture per cookie cutter.

Finally, coat the tops with cooking spray and start baking them at 475 degrees Fahrenheit. Let them stay there for 20 minutes before turning them over, this time for another 15 minute cooking time.

Dinner

Bean Burger

A little exhaustive but nonetheless a great find, this Bean Burger recipe may be perfect for you!

- ½ cup water
- 3 tbsp of extra virgin olive oil
- ¼ cup quinoa
- 1 clove minced garlic
- ½ cup of red onion, chopped
- 1 tsp of smoked paprika
- 2.5 cup of pinto beans, cooked
- ½ tsp salt
- 3 tbsp of cornmeal and 1/3 cup for coating the burger
- Freshly ground pepper
- ½ tsp of cumin seeds, grounded and toasted
- 3 tbsp of fresh cilantro, chopped
- 6 whole-wheat hamburger buns
- 6 tomato slices
- 6 lettuce leaves
- 2 tbsp of fresh cilantro, freshly chopped
- 1 avocado, ripe
- 1 tbsp of lemon juice
- 1 clove of garlic, minced
- 2 tbsp of red onion, finely chopped
- 1/5 tsp of salt
- 1/5 tsp of cayenne pepper

You'll notice that some ingredients seem to be doubled – for a very good reason. You'll be using them several times throughout the recipe so try to divide them beforehand. Here's how to work on this delicious burger:

- Start by boiling water in a saucepan and tossing in the quinoa which should take about 10 minutes. Lower the heat a few minutes in until all the water is absorbed.
- Grab a skillet and put in ½ cup of onion and garlic for around 3 minutes. Pour in the beans, the paprika, and the cumin.
- Mash the beans until you create a thick paste. Allow it to cool for a few minutes before adding the quinoa and mixing in 3 tsp of cornmeal, 3 tbsp of cilantro, and ½ tsp of salt and pepper. Stir them thoroughly. This is your main patty so mash them together and create decent sized burger patty. Coat the patty with some cornmeal.
- Line them in a baking sheet and refrigerate for 30 minutes so that they'd retain their shape.

The rest of the ingredients are for creating guacamole. Here's what to do:

- Start by mashing the avocado together and adding in the lemon juice, 2tsp of onion, cayenne, garlic, and 2 tbsp of cilantro. Add some cayenne and salt to taste.
- By this time, your patties should be ready. Preheat the oven to 200 degrees Fahrenheit and grab your patties from the fridge.
- Grab a skillet and put in some oil over medium heat. Cook the burgers in it until they get that brown and crisp coloring.
- Once done, put them inside the oven to keep them crispy warm.
- Put in toasted buns and serve with guacamole on the side. They're perfect together with hash browns!

Halibut, Ginger, and Green Onions

A little extensive when it comes to ingredients, this particular recipe is something you can cook for those special nights when you have the luxury of a long and relaxing bath afterwards.

Ingredients are as follows:

- 4 halibut fillets – although you can exchange them for lean meat
- ¼ tsp pepper
- 1 tbsp gingerroot, peeled and minced
- 1/8 tsp salt
- 1 tbsp fresh lime juice
- 2 tsp grazed lime zest
- 1 garlic clove, medium and minced
- 1 tbsp soy sauce, low sodium
- ¼ cup green onions, thinly sliced
- 1/8 tsp toasted sesame oil
- 2 tsp canola or corn oil
- 1 tsp canola or corn oil

Start by sprinkling some salt and pepper onto the fish, spreading them around to distribute the taste. Cook the fish in a non-stick skillet coated by just 2 teaspoons of canola oil using medium heat. Wait 2 minutes and then flip the fish, cooking the other side in the same amount of time. Once done, set the fish aside.

Load one teaspoon of canola oil into the same skillet and start cooking the green onion, ginger, and garlic until you get that amazing aroma. Remove it from the heat and pour in all the other ingredients remaining. Stir them all together and spoon them over your halibut.

Cabbage Rolls

A mouthwatering combination of protein and fiber, these cabbage rolls are best made for dinner since they take a long time to cook. They're worth it though!

Here's an ingredient list:

- ½ cup of brown rice
- 3 pounds Savoy cabbage
- 1 cup water
- 1 onion, medium sized and chopped
- 1 tbsp canola oil
- 6 tbsp lemon juice
- 1 pound lean ground turkey
- 4 cloves of minced garlic
- 1 tsp caraway seeds
- ½ tsp salt
- ½ tsp pepper, freshly ground
- 3 tbsp fresh dill, chopped
- 1 tbsp honey
- 1 cup chicken broth, reduced sodium
- 1 ½ cup tomato salt, without salt

Start by cooking the rice first. You can do this by combining the brown rice with the water for 25 to 35 minutes. Reduce the heat around the 20-minute mark since cooking rice can be tricky. Once the rice is soft and fluffy, you should remove it from the heat and allow it to cool down.

Start working on the cabbage leaves by boiling the largest ones in water for 6 minutes. The rest of the cabbages can be chopped into small pieces and used for something else later.

Taking a saucepan, start adding some oil into it and after properly heated; add the chopped cabbage and the onion. Stir often until they're soft. Add in the garlic and around 4 tablespoons of lemon juice. Stir slowly with the heat kept low until the liquid is all gone. Set it aside and allow cooling.

Preheat the oven to 375 degrees Fahrenheit

Now grab the turkey and mix it together with pepper, caraway, salt, and dill. Add in the rice and the onion mixture into the bowl and stir.

Grab a pan and coat it with some cooking spray. Grab a cabbage leaf and put some turkey mixture inside, essentially creating a 'roll' by folding the leaves together and closing it with a toothpick. Line them on the pan and bake for one hour.

You have the option of basting the rolls in between cooking with a mixture of tomato sauce, honey, broth, and cabbage leaves. You can also freeze a batch of the turkey mixture so that you can create more in the following days without consuming as much time in the process.

Fish and Chips – Oven Cooked

Come dinner, you should have more time to leisurely prepare food and enjoy a full course meal. Oven cooked fish and chips should be a healthy way to end the day. Here's how to do it:

For ingredients, you'd want the following:

- Olive oil cooking spray
- 4 tsp of canola oil
- 2 cups cornflakes
- 1 ½ tsp of Creole seasoning
- ¼ pound of russet potatoes cut into wedges
- 1/4 tsp salt
- 2 large eggs, use the white only and beat it to a thick froth

- ¼ cup all purpose flour
- 1 pound cod

This should take only about 1 hour and 30 minutes in all.

- Start by preheating the oven to 425 degrees Fahrenheit
- Coat the baking sheet and wire rack with cooking spray. Place the wire rack on a different baking sheet so you'd have two: one without the wire rack and another with a wire rack.
- Wash the potatoes and make sure they're completely dry. Toss them into a mixture of ¾ Creole and oil.
- Spread the potatoes on the plain baking sheet and start baking them in the oven. Make sure they're in the lower rack and turn them every 10 minutes until they're tender and gold in color. This should take around 30 minutes and the chips are done!

For the fish, this is what you have to do:

- Grind some cornflakes by crushing them in a plastic bag or use a food processor if you want a wine result. Set them aside.
- Combine the following: ¾ of Creole, flour, egg white, salt and seasonings. Don't go overboard with the salt since this is a known trigger for hypertension. In fact, if you can skip the salt entirely – that would be perfect.
- Dip the fish in the liquid mixture and use the cornflakes to cover the wet fish in it for that very crunchy feel after cooking.
- Put them in the wire rack and bake for 20 minutes. Use the upper portion of the oven rack.

Snacks and Shakes

Let's say you don't have the time to do all those – but you do have the time to prepare a light snack. Here are some of the snacks-slash-meals that you can prepare:

Yogurt and Orange

Add these ingredients together in a blender and enjoy!

- ¾ cup low-fat yogurt, plain
- 2 tbsp of nonfat dry milk
- ½ cup of orange juice
- 1 tbsp of honey
- ½ tsp of vanilla extract
- 1 tbsp of toasted wheat germ

Banana, Cocoa, and Soy

It might seem like an icky combination at first- but you might be surprised at how good it tastes! Combine the following:

- 1 banana
- ½ cup soymilk
- ½ cup silken tofu
- 1 tbsp honey
- 2 tbsp unsweetened cocoa powder

Try to keep the bananas in the freezer overnight to get that smooth and cool blend. This also helps the banana stay longer.

Blueberry and Bananas

To make 4 servings of this drink, add the following and blend:

- 2 ripe banana
- Frozen blueberries, 2 cups
- Baby spinach, 2 cups
- Non fat yogurt, 2 cups

Since this would make 4 glasses, you can try decreasing the amount so that you only get 1 or 2 glasses in one blending session. Keep in mind that freshly made smoothies are best so make sure you're not going to keep it in the fridge for later. If you decide to do this though, smoothies will keep overnight – but they won't be as satisfying.

Smoothie Parfait

A little tough to make thanks to the multiple blender rinsing you have to do, this smoothie parfait is at least guaranteed to be delicious. Here are the ingredients:

- ½ cup of unsweetened blueberries
- 2 tbsp of frozen acai pulp
- ½ tbsp of cold water
- ½ tsp agave nectar
- ½ cup cubed ripe mango
- ¼ cup of ice
- 1 tbsp of toasted wheat germ
- 1 tbsp of fresh lime juice
- 2 tbsp of flaked unsweetened coconut
- ½ cup unsweetened pineapple cubes
- ¼ cup coconut water

Start by putting the blueberries, acai pulp, agave nectar, and cold water in a blender and mixing them all together. Set aside in a chilled glass, rinse, and blend again these particular ingredients: lime juice, ice, and wheat germ. When smooth, spoon the blueberry mixture inside. Last, put in all the other remaining ingredient in the blender after rinsing it. Spoon them into the chilled glass and enjoy!

Vanilla Latte

This is something you can order through many stores. Just ask the server to use soymilk for your latte instead of regular milk. If they don't have soymilk, you can always order non-fat milk.

Fruit Salsa

A fruit platter is always great if you want to feast on all the flavors nature has to offer. If you want to kick it up a notch however, you can always add some onions, cilantro, and lime to the fruit platter for that extra amazing taste.

Jamie's Easy Granola

This recipe shared by health.com lets you create granola bars quickly and easily. The great thing about making large batches of granola bars is that you can just grab them for a quick lunch and dinner, knowing that you're getting enough vitamins and minerals each time.

Here's what you'll need:

- 2 cups of oatmeal, the non-instant kind
- ¼ cup of mixed seeds
- 1 cup mixed nuts
- 1 tsp of ground cinnamon
- ¾ cup of unsweetened shredded coconut

- 1 ½ cups dried fruit
- 3 tbsp of olive oil
- 5 tbsp of maple syrup

Start by preheating the oven to 350 degrees Fahrenheit and mix together all the dry ingredients together with the oatmeal. Stir well before drizzling in the maple syrup and olive oil. Once done, bake the whole thing for 25 minutes. Try to remove it from the oven every few minutes just to stir the mixture and make sure every single portion is cooked. Remove and allow it to cool down before serving. You can keep any leftovers in an airtight container and eat them for quick nourishments. Properly saved, they can last up to 2 weeks!

Food Substitution

Of course, having high blood pressure doesn't mean you can't eat your favorite fares anymore. For the most part, lowering your salt intake means simply altering your favorite recipes to keep the sodium and other unhealthy ingredients away from your daily intake. Hence, you can always choose to use food substitutes so that you can still enjoy cooking favorites without all salt. Here are some ideal substitutes for certain food items:

Soy Sauce and Teriyaki Sauce Substitute - Molasses

If you're a fan of this Asian sauce you might want to step back a notch and opt for lower-sodium counterparts for your recipe. Fortunately, you can rely on molasses to help save the taste while keeping your sodium levels within the normal range. It's often included with rice-wine vinegar to get that teriyaki-sauce taste that you're craving for sushi or dumplings.

Bread Substitute – Tacos

We've probably mentioned how bread is one of the biggest sodium culprits known today. It's not surprising considering how sodium is used as a preservative and bread has to last as long as possible on the shelves. While you can check out low-sodium bread, you can also opt for healthier alternatives. There are tacos shells that offer the same taste without the salt. You can also try using cabbage leaves instead of bread, as shown in the Cabbage Rolls recipe.

Milk Substitute – Coconut Milk

While milk is an excellent dairy product that sort of helps with high blood pressure; too much is not really a good idea. So what do you do? You use coconut milk to get the same amazing taste for your recipe without the obvious sodium content. Coconut milk can be a substitute for practically all kinds of cooked dishes as well as the non-cooked ones. For example, you might want to switch whole milk for coconut milk in your cereal or coffee!

Broth Substitute – Mushroom Broth

Ditch the typical broth and use mushroom as your base for stew and other recipes requiring thick and tasty broth. This offers the earthy flavor of umami which adds a whole new dimension to your cooking. While it's not exactly salty, it has this unique feel that turns your cooking rich and addictive.

Of course, there are always low sodium alternatives in the market today. Just keep in mind that the sodium content should be checked out before you buy the stuff. Do the math if necessary to make sure that your sodium is within the daily recommended amount.

Chapter 9: Living With High Blood Pressure - Eating Out

The general rule is to avoid eating out as much as possible since you never really know what's involved in cooking these food items. Of course, there are instances when you can't help but order something from the restaurant because of time constraints. Here are some ideas on what to order to keep your diet low in sodium:

Starbucks Oatmeal

Yup – Starbucks offers healthy oatmeal but with a few tweaks on your part. You can ask your Starbucks server to use nonfat milk or soymilk for your oatmeal. You can also skip the nuts, raisins, and brown sugar because they add fat to the meal. If you must however – make sure to use the packets sparingly and just save the rest for snacks later. Other Starbucks stores offer additional fruits like blueberries and banana so you might want to get those and just slice them into the oatmeal.

Subway Veggie Sandwich

Subway can create something that's good for your blood pressure – but only if you ask them to do so. The regular Subway fare is a little too much so here's what you have to do. Start by having the bread scooped out and then load it with lettuce, tomatoes, pepper, spinach, cucumbers, and every other kind of veggie you feel like eating. Dairy is good but keep it limited. Avocado is also helpful but keeps in mind that avocados are packed with calories. As to olives – skip them entirely since they're often soaked in sodium. Your spread would be vinegar and mustard with some sprinklings of oregano and black pepper.

Salad Bar

A salad bar can be found in practically any and all supermarkets or chain stores. If you're lucky enough to be located near one, take advantage of their wonderful offerings as well as the convenience of having your lunch in as little as 15 minutes. Since they're all vegetables – there's really no stopping you from choosing and eating as much as you want. Just remember that you dressing should be confined to balsamic vinegar or something fat free.

Wendy's Baked Potatoes

Potatoes aren't usually favored for a high blood pressure diet – but that's because most people eat them fried. French fries and fried potato wedges are not good for people with hypertension. If you bake them however, they become excellent fares to keep that pressure down. Wendy's has excellent baked potato which should help trim the waist while keeping your blood pressure within normal levels. Bear in mind though that you should steer clear of any high calorie toppings like sour cream and butter. Instead, opt for the pico de gallo topping which Wendy's also serves.

Side Garden Salad from Burger King

No need to have anything altered – just request for this particular meal with the avocado ranch dressing and you're good to go. This meal contains just 540 mg worth of sodium and calories of just 240 so it's perfect for those who are trying to lose weight.

Traditional Wings from Pizza Hut

Who doesn't love the traditional wings from Pizza Hut with their mouth watering taste? Packed with protein – it's easy to fall in love with this meal, especially since it contains only 290 mg worth of sodium. The calories are also just 80 in all, but keep in mind that moderation is still the key.

Wendy's Garden Side Salad with Light Honey and French Dressing

Another offering from Wendy's, this salad contains just 115mg of sodium and according to the website, just 60 calories.

McDonald's Premium Southwest Salad

This contains just 150mg worth of sodium – but bear in mind that this is without the chicken. Total calories are approximately 140mg.

McDonald's Fruit and Yogurt Parfait

Fruit and yogurt typically have low sodium – but you can't expect much when it comes from McDonalds. Just be glad that this particular health choice contains just 70mg worth of sodium with calories of just 150.

Additional Tips

- Not everyone has the privilege of having the restaurant chef customize the food according to their diet. If you're one of the lucky few however, make sure your chef knows that you're on a low-sodium diet and thus, your meal should be reduced in sodium.
- Always ask for the dressing on the side rather than splendidly spread around your salad. This way, you can easily control how much of this sodium-packed gets added onto your daily allowance.

Conclusion

Once diagnosed with high blood pressure, it's often a good idea to check your BP every now and then just to make sure that you're not beyond the normal range.

You'll find that having an electronic BP can work wonders in making sure you remain within normal levels even without visiting a doctor. There are also apps today that let you check up on your blood pressure without having to buy a specific product to get the same results.

Remember: controlling your BP requires a lifestyle change and not just a single substitution in your daily life! Change your diet, get some exercise, reduce stress, and get some sleep – all of these are factors into giving you a healthy BP!

Lastly, if you enjoyed reading the book, could you please take time to share your views with us by posting a review on Amazon? Having a positive review from you helps the book reach many more people, so we can continue to reach those who can benefit from the information shared within the book. It'd be highly appreciated!

Congratulations to your new, healthy, low blood pressure life!

Blood Pressure Solution

54 Delicious Heart Healthy Recipes that will Naturally Lower High Blood Pressure and Reduce Hypertension

Introduction

Congratulations on purchasing your very own copy of *Blood Pressure Solution*. Thank you so much for doing so!

This book will discuss one of the most probable causes of death in America today: the rise of blood pressure levels. Blood pressure plays a big role in keeping our bodies at a healthy and maintained level for survival. Decreases and increases in this variable can cause major health complications down the road, but I am here to inform you that you can fix it by making small changes in your diet!

The contents of this book are filled with valuable information that will help support you in your journey of lowering your blood pressure by your next doctor appointment! You will discover that what you consume is the major cause of why your blood pressure is higher than it should be.

Each of the recipes tucked away within the chapters of this book are designed to keep you on the straight and narrow as you get your blood pressure under control, all while not sacrificing taste and satisfaction! Each recipe includes the components needs to prepare them, preparation times, nutritional facts and one of the most important factors in rising blood pressure: sodium levels.
Enjoy your journey through the pages of this recipe book as you discover more information about your health and delicious eats to try in the comfort of your own home! Good luck!

There are plenty of books regarding blood pressure on the market, so thanks again for choosing this one! Every effort was made to ensure it is full of as much useful information as possible. Please enjoy!

The Dangers of a Rising Blood Pressure

High blood pressure is something that can plague the body for many years without a person realizing it. Also referred to as hypertension, its symptoms, if left uncontrolled, can cause one to develop a disability, death by heart attack or a poor quality of the remainder of life a person has. There are many complications that come with a high blood pressure count. But fortunately, this book is here to bring to light that a change in diet alone can help to decrease your overall blood pressure immensely!

Complications of Hypertension

Destruction of the arteries

Arteries that are healthy are strong and elastic in nature. The inner lining within them is smooth so that the blood flowing through them can flow freely through them, providing vital organs and tissues within the body with oxygen and proper nutrients. Over time, hypertension increases the amount of blood flowing through your arteries. Because of this, you may have to deal with these health issues:

- *Narrowed and damaged arteries* – High blood pressure damages cells that make up the inner lining that inhibits the arteries. When fats that you consume enter into the blood stream, they have a tendency to collect in the damaged arteries, causing them to become much less elastic which results in a limit of blood flow throughout the entirety of the body.

- *Aneurysm* – A constant heightened amount of blood moving through weakened arteries can have the potential to cause enlargements within artery walls that result in the development of an aneurysm. These bad fellas can explode and result in terrible ailments that can harm your entire life, such as bleeding internally. Aneurysms develop within the arteries in the body, but they tend to be found most often right within the aorta, known as the biggest artery in our bodies.

Deterioration of the heart

Your heart is the organ responsible for getting blood to your entire body. The presence of hypertension will result in exponential damage to your heart in numerous ways, such as:

- *Heart failure* – The strain on your heart over time that is caused by hypertension will cause the muscles in your heart to weaken, causing it to not work near as efficiently as it's supposed to. Your heart will become overwhelmed, eventually wearing out and failing. Damage from heart attacks that are also caused by high blood pressure will only add to this serious issue.

- *Enlarged left heart* – The presence of hypertension forces the heart to pump harder and more often than it usually does in order to get the required blood to all areas of your body. This will cause your left ventricle of your heart become rather stiff over time, which is known as left ventricular hypertrophy. This then inhibits your ventricle's job of being able to pump blood as efficiently as it is supposed to. This condition will increase your risk of having a heart attack, congestive heart failure and even cardiac death that can arise out of nowhere rather suddenly.

- *Coronary artery disease* – This disease affects your arteries that are responsible for providing blood right to the core of your heart muscles. Arteries become narrowed over time, which does not allow blood to flow as freely as it should throughout the arteries in your body. As a result, a person with coronary artery disease can experience irregular heart rhythms, heart attack and varying degrees of chest pain.

Damage to your brain

Your brain, just like your heart, is another crucial organ within your body that heavily relies on a constant flow of nourishing blood supply in order for it to work properly. High blood pressure can cause several issues within your noggin, like:

- *Mild cognitive impairment* – This ailment is a just the stage that lies in-between understanding all the changes that happen to one's memory when natural aging occurs and the point at which those are more susceptible to developing diseases such as Alzheimer's. Like other brain ailments, it can be caused by blocked blood flow to the brain.

- *Dementia* – This is a disease that lives within the brain that impairs normal and necessary human functions such as movement, vision, memory, reasoning, speaking, and thinking. There are a few causes that result in dementia. Vascular dementia is a result of the narrowing of arteries and the blockage within them that keeps an adequate blood supply from flowing to the brain.

- *Stroke* – Strokes happen when part of the brain becomes deprived of nutrients and oxygen, which results in the death of brain cells. High blood pressure that is uncontrolled can lead to a stroke because it damages and majorly weakens the blood vessels in your brain, resulting in them becoming narrowed, rupturing and leaking. Hypertension is also the culprit behind the development of blood clots within the arteries that directly trail the way to the brain, blocking proper blood flow and potentially causing someone to have a stroke.

- *Transient ischemic attack*– Also referred to as a mini-stroke, these attacks are very brief, due to a disruption of blood flow to the brain. It is a direct cause as a result of atherosclerosis (blood clot) which can develop from having high blood pressure. IF you have one of these attacks, you should view it as a big red flag that you may be at major risk for experiencing a full-blown stroke later down the road.

Damage to your kidneys

Your kidneys are the organ in the body that filters out other fluids that are excess and other wastes from your blood. This process is dependent on having healthy blood vessels. The presence of hypertension will lead to these vital blood vessels becoming damaged, which can then result in you developing several forms of kidney disease. The damage has the potential to be much worse in those with diabetes.

- *Kidney failure* – High blood pressure takes the gold as being one of the most popular causes for the result of kidney failure. Hypertension can damage not only the larger arteries that lead to your kidneys but also the tiny blood vessels that live within your kidneys as well. Both are crucial to a thriving life. Damage to either of these can cause your kidneys to not be fully capable of filtering waste from your body. This puts the body at risk, for wastes accumulate over time and you may have to undergo dialysis or kidney transplant.

- *Kidney scarring* – Also known as glomerulosclerosis, kidney scarring is a type of kidney damage that occurs to the glomeruli, which are mini clusters made if vessels living within your kidneys that are responsible for filtering fluids and wastes from your blood. This can leave your kidneys with the lack of capability to filter wastes effectively, which can lead to kidney failure.

- *Kidney artery aneurysm* – Aneurysms are bulges that live within the walls of vessels that occur over time. This particular type of aneurysms takes place in the artery that leads to your kidneys. High blood pressure, over time, will weaken this artery and cause sections to become enlarged and form bulges. Aneurysms can rupture and threaten the life of those who have them with internal bleeding.

Disturbances of the eyes

There are many tiny and very intricate blood vessels that provide necessary blood to that of your eyes. Just like all vessels within the body, they have the potential to become damaged over time, especially if the presence of high blood pressure wreaks havoc on your body.

- *Eye blood vessel damage* – Also referred to as retinopathy, it is caused directly by hypertension damaged the blood vessels that supply your retinas with blood. This can cause conditions like bleeding of eyes, blurred vision and at the very worst, complete vision loss. If one has diabetes and hypertension, they are at a much greater risk of developing these conditions.

- *Buildup of fluid underneath the retina(s)* – Also known as choroidopathy, this occurs when the buildup of fluid happens underneath your retina(s) due to a blood vessel (or blood vessels) that may have burst and are leaking under the retina itself. This condition can result in a major distortion of vision and even has the potential to scar your eyes, which can lead to impaired vision.

- *Nerve damage* – Also referred to as optic neuropathy, this condition results from a blockage in blood flow that damages the optic nerve. It is responsible for killing off nerve cells within the eyes, which can result in bleeding in the eyes and potential for vision loss.

Sexual dysfunction

Although ailments such as erectile dysfunction and other such medical conditions that inhibit proper sexual functions can occur as a result of aging, the presence of high blood pressure can drastically increase the likelihood of developing these sorts of conditions. Over time, hypertension damages the lining of the vessels within these areas of your body, which will mean less blood flow to the penis and vagina, which leads to the incapability of maintaining an erection and a decreased desire in sexual intercourse. Women can also have vaginal dryness and difficulty achieving orgasms.

Bone Loss

High blood pressure has the potential to increase calcium amounts and deposits within the urine. With this major decrease of calcium from the body, these are a direct result of a loss of overall bone density which can lead to breaking more bones. The risks of osteoporosis are seen more often in women.

Trouble Sleeping

With those with high blood pressure issues, a condition known as obstructive sleep apnea can occur. This condition causes the relaxation of your throat muscles, which can lead to excessive snoring. While it has been shown that hypertension itself can directly trigger sleep apnea, sleep deprivation as a result of this condition also can be a trigger as well.

Symptoms of High Blood Pressure

Hypertension can at times be hard to detect because many people live for a long time with little to no symptoms or warning signs. This means that people do not feel like they need to go to the doctor and get anything checked out, which is why so many seemingly healthy individuals suffer from the long-term effects of hypertension later on. It is important to not take these symptoms of hypertension lightly:

- Shortness of breath
- Dizziness
- Blurred vision
- Headache

Things that Raise your Blood Pressure

High blood pressure is determined by a set of numbers; the first number is 140 or higher or if the second number is 90 or higher. There are many circumstances that physicians don't know what directly causes hypertension. It is said that family history, your age and your race all have the potential to play a factor. But these things are proven to be direct causes in the development of high blood pressure:

- *Too much salt* – Sodium is known for raising your blood pressure because it plays a major role in the narrowing of your vessels within your body that enables your body to hold on to more fluid. It is best to limit the amount of salt you consume. Alongside this rule, you need to eat plenty of potassium so that you have a fighting chance to successfully balance your sodium levels and keep high blood pressure at bay.

- *Lack of exercise* - When you spend most of your time on the couch binge watching Orange is the New Black and other shows all day; you are putting yourself in danger of a rising heart rate, which makes the heart work much harder than it needs to. But during the course of the exercise, hormones in the body relax your blood vessels and help to lower blood pressure levels.
- *Being overweight* – When you weight goes up, so does the amount of blood you need to flow to the growing portions of your body. This puts more strain directly on your heart which results in your blood vessels picking up the slack. This is why a good balance of physical activity and a healthy diet are so vital to keeping your hypertension at bay.

- *Tobacco use* – Smoking cigarettes and chewing tobacco both raise your blood pressure levels. Chemicals within these products damage your vessels which then narrows them, leading them to develop hypertension.

- *Alcohol use* – Consuming alcohol heavily on a regular basis can majorly damage your heart muscles. This is why you should limit your alcohol intake.

- *Stress* – Large amounts of stress or chronic stress can cause issues with blood pressure. It leads to starting bad habits such as smoking and drinking which as you have read, are neither the best at keeping your blood pressure levels low.

As you have read, having high blood pressure has no perks! Whether you are dedicated to living a healthier lifestyle to avoid these health issues caused by hypertension later on, or you are already struggling with problems because of your blood pressure levels, the remainder of this book is filled with recipes that will aid you in your mission to lower those threatening levels! There is no need for your taste buds to suffer in order for you to be a healthier individual! That's dive into the wide array of delicious recipes, shall we?

Breakfast Recipes

During the course of the night Chia Oatmeal

Preparation time: 5 min.

Complete time: 8 hours – During the course of the night

Calories 289 – Carbs 23g – Sodium 3g – Fat 9g

What's in it:

- ¼ tsp. nutmeg
- ¼ tsp. ground ginger
- ¼ tsp. vanilla extract
- ¼ tsp. cinnamon
- ¼ tsp. ground cardamom
- 2 tbsp. shredded coconut
- 2 tbsp. chia seeds
- 1 C. coconut almond milk
- 1 C. oats

How it's made:

- Combine all components in a medium sized bowl. Top the bowl with wrap, preferably plastic.
- Frost for 8 hours or during the course of the night. (It is much better during the course of the night!)

Sarah's Easy Homemade Applesauce

Preparation time: Ten to fifteen min.

Complete time: An hour

Calories 309 – Carbs 12g – Sodium 2.5g – Fat 11g

What's in it:

- ½ tsp. ground cinnamon
- ¼ C. white sugar
- ¾ C. water
- 4 apples - peeled, cored and chopped

How it's made:

- Mix together all components in a saucepan.
- Cook covered over intermediate to immense warmth 15 into 20 min. until apples become tender.
- Let apples sit and cool and proceed to mash with a potato masher or fork.

Egg Scramble

Preparation time: 15 min.
Complete time: 40 min.

Calories 270 – Carbs 12g – Sodium 3g – Fat 11.2g

What's in it:

- ¼ C. cheddar cheese, shredded
- A sprinkle of hot pepper sauce
- Ground cayenne
- Pepper and salt
- 2 seeded and chopped tomatoes
- 4 beaten eggs
- ½ C. freshly chopped spinach
- 2 cloves of garlic, chopped
- 1 chopped onion
- 1 peeled potato

How it's made:

- Get out a small pot. Put water in it with a few dashes of salt and heat to boiling point.
- Pour in the potato and cook for 15 min. until it is tenderized yet still firm. Remove liquid, let it cool and cut up potato.
- Sauté garlic and onion in a skillet over intermediate to immense warmth.
- Then, proceed to add in spinach, cooking it until it's wilted, around 2 min.
- Decrease your heat to medium and put in eggs. Cook for 2 min. until the bottom is set.
- Mix in tomatoes and potatoes, sprinkling with salt,

pepper, and cayenne as desired. Add in hot sauce as well.

- Stir mixture occasionally until the eggs are set.
- Sprinkle your scrambled eggs with grated cheese. Serve warm!

Beer Batter Crepes

Preparation time: 5 min.
Complete time: 10-15 min.

Calories 302 – Carbs 9g – Sodium 2.2g – Fat 9g

What's in it:

- 2 tbsp. butter
- 2 tbsp. vegetable oil
- A pinch of salt
- 1 ¾ C. regular white flour
- 1 C. beer
- 1 C. milk
- 3 lightly beaten eggs

How it's made:

- Whisk beer, eggs, and milk.
- Then gradually mix in the flour.
- Pour in salt and oil, then combine mixture rapidly three to five min., so everything is well mixed. Allow the batter sit for at least 1 hour.
- Over intermediate to immense warmth, heat a 10" skillet. Brush with butter.
- Once skillet is hot but not yet smoking, pour one-third of a cup of the mixture into the central area of cooking pan you are using, ensuring batter covers the entirety of the bottom of your skillet. Make sure to pour out the excess batter before continuing to cook.
- Cook crepe 1 to 2 min. until it becomes golden in color.
- Then, flip it over and cook other side for 30 seconds.
- Put on a plate covered in foil to ensure they are kept

toasty as you continue cooking the remaining crepes.

- Continue above process until batter is all used.
- Fill with fruit, veggies or anything else you desire!

Sausage Egg Muffins

Preparation time: 10 to 15 min.
Complete time: 30 to 40 min.

Calories 299 – Carbs 11g – Sodium 5g – Fat 14g

What's in it:

- Pepper and salt
- 1 tsp. garlic powder
- 1 chopped onion
- ½ can of chopped green chili peppers
- 12 beaten eggs
- ½ pound low-sodium ground sausage

How it's made:

- Ensure that your oven is preheated to 350 degrees.
- Lightly grease some muffin cups or a muffin tin.
- In a deep skillet on intermediate to immense warmth, place sausage and cook until browned. Remove liquid and then set to the side.
- Combine all the components and sausage in a large bowl until well mixed.
- Spoon ¼ cup of the mixture into each of the muffin cups.
- Bake 15 to 20 min. until the egg has set and a toothpick put into the middle of muffins turns out with no more batter upon it.

Ultimate Irresistible Granola

Preparation time: 10 min.
Complete time: 30 min.

Calories 312 – Carbs 11g – Sodium 2g – Fat 8g

What's in it:

- 1 C. dried cranberries
- 1 C. raisins
- 1 ½ C. honey
- 1 C. canola oil
- 1 C. unsalted sunflower seeds
- 2 C. coconut, shredded
- 1 C. wheat germ
- 1 C. sesame seeds
- 1 C. pecans cut up
- 1 C. walnuts cut up
- 1 C. blanched slivered almonds
- 5 C. rolled oats

How it's made:

- Ensure oven is preheated to 325 degrees.
- Mix together sunflower seeds, coconut, wheat germ, sesame seeds, pecans, walnuts, almonds and oats in a bowl.
- Over intermediate to immense warmth, stir together honey and oil in a pan. Cook until blended.
- Pour honey batter over oat mixture and stir up thoroughly.
- Put batter out on 2 cookie sheets.
- Back each for 20 min. until oats and nuts are toasted.

- Once it comes out of the oven, stir in cranberries and raisins.
- Let cook and stir again in order to break up large clusters.
- Store in airtight container for 2 weeks. Enjoy!

Banana Bran Muffins

Preparation time: 20 min.
Complete time: 45 min.

Calories 256 – Carbs 17g – Sodium 4g – Fat 8.9g

What's in it:

- ¼ tsp. salt
- ½ tsp. cinnamon
- ½ tsp. baking soda
- 1 ½ tsp. baking powder
- ¾ C. regular white flour
- 1 C. whole wheat flour
- 1 tsp. vanilla extract
- ¼ C. canola oil
- 1 C. unprocessed wheat bran
- 1 C. buttermilk
- 1 C. mashed ripe bananas
- 2/3 C. packed light brown sugar
- ½ C. chocolate chips (optional)
- 1/3 C. chopped walnuts (optional)

How it's made:

- Ensure your oven is preheated until it reaches 400 degrees.
- Grease up your muffin cups or a muffin tin with greasing medium of choice.
- Mix brown sugar and eggs together, then adding in buttermilk, bananas, wheat bran, vanilla, and oil.

- In another vessel that is bowl shaped, mix together salt, cinnamon, baking soda, baking powder, and flours until combined.
- Create a divot in your dry ingredient mixture and add in wet components, stirring until mixed and smooth. Stir in chocolate chips if you have decided to use them.
- Spoon batter into muffin tins (will be full) and top with walnuts.
- Bake 15 to 25 min. until muffins are visibly golden and when you put a finger gently among the top it springs back at you.
- Allow to sit 5 min., undo edges with a butter knife and set the muffin on a rack made of wire to let cool for a few more min. before you eat. Yum!

Wake Up Smoothie

Preparation Time: 5 min.

Calories 139 – Carbs 28g – Sodium 10g – Fat 2g

What's in it:

- 1 tbsp. Splenda
- ½ C. low-fat tofu or low-fat plain yogurt
- 1 ¼ C. frozen berries of choice
- 1 banana
- 1 ¼ C. orange juice (recommended: calcium-fortified)

How it's made:

- Combine all components until smooth and creamy in a blender.
- Serve right away as a great breakfast treat to start off your day right!

Cinnamon Bake Donuts

Preparation time: 15 min.
Complete time: 35 min.

Calories 210 – Carbs 13g – Sodium 5g – Fat 9g

What's in it:

- 2 tsp. pure vanilla extract
- 2 tbsp. unsalted butter, melted
- 1 ¼ C. whole milk
- 1 large lightly beaten egg
- ½ tsp. salt
- ½ tsp. nutmeg
- 1 tsp. cinnamon
- 2 tsp. baking powder
- 1 ½ C. sugar
- Spray for greasing

Topping:

- ½ tsp. ground cinnamon
- ½ C. sugar
- 8 tbsp. unsalted butter

How it's made:

- Ensure oven is preheated to 350 degrees. Sprays a couple of donut pans well with greasing medium of choice.
- Sift salt, nutmeg, cinnamon, baking powder, sugar, and flour together.
- In a small bowl, stir vanilla, melted butter and egg

together well.

- Pour and mix in wet mixture into dry components and combine.
- Pour your mixture into baking pans, filling each a bit more than ¾ of the way full.
- Bake 17 min., until a toothpick turns out with no batter on it.
- Let cool for at least 5 min., then put donuts on top of a sheet pan.
- *For topping:* Within a sauté pan, melt your butter. Mix together cinnamon and sugar. Set to the side for a minute.
- Dip each donut in the butter and proceed to emerge each one in cinnamon-sugar. You can sugar up one or both sides. Indulge!

French Toast

Preparation time: 20 min.
Complete time: 30 min.

Calories 260 – Carbs 20g – Sodium 11g – Fat 9.8g
What's in it:

- ½ C. warmed maple syrup
- 8 slices of white, brioche or challah bread
- ½ tsp. vanilla extract
- ¼ C. milk
- 4 eggs
- 4 tbsp. butter
- 2 tbsp. sugar
- ¼ tsp. nutmeg
- 1 tsp. ground cinnamon

How it's made:

- Combine sugar, nutmeg, and cinnamon. Set to the side.
- In a pan over intermediate to immense warmth, melt butter.
- Whisk cinnamon mixture, vanilla, milk, and eggs together and pour into a shallow container.
- Dip bread in egg mixture.
- Fry slices of bread until they are a light golden brown hue.
- Eat with warm maple syrup.

Breakfast Power Balls

Preparation time: 20 min.
Complete time: 1 hour and 20 min.

Calories 157 – Carbs 11g – Sodium 6g – Fat 19g

What's in it:

- 2 tbsp. flax seed
- ½ C. unsalted sunflower seeds
- ½ C. dried cranberries
- ½ C. mini chocolate chips
- ½ C. raw honey
- 1 C. extra-crunchy peanut butter
- 2 C. rolled oats

How it's made:

- Pulse together flax seeds, sunflower seeds, cranberries, chocolate chips, honey, peanut butter and oats in a food processor until combined. Cover and Frost for 30 min.
- With waxed paper, line a baking sheet. Form balls from the mixture and place them on the sheet. Frost for 30 min. before consuming.

Frozen Fruit Cups

Complete time: 10 min.

Calories 123 – Carbs 5g – Sodium 2g – Fat 5g

What's in it:

- 1/3 C. lemon juice
- 1 small can of frozen pineapple-orange juice concentrate (thawed)
- 6 chopped bananas
- 1 can fruit cocktail (liquid removed)
- 2 cans crushed pineapple (liquid removed)
- 2 cans mandarin oranges (liquid removed)
- 4 C. frozen peaches (thawed and chopped)

How it's made:

- Mix all components of the recipe together in a bowl until combined.
- Place fruit mixture into plastic disposable cups, covering with plastic wrap.
- Freeze until firm.
- Remove from freezer 45 min. to an hour before you wish to serve to give time for fruit cups to thaw enough to thoroughly enjoy.

Vanilla Bean Coconut Yogurt Smoothie

Preparation time: 5 min.
Complete time: 27 min.

Calories 101 – Carbs 5g – Sodium 4g – Fat 9g

What's in it:

- Coconut water (frozen in ice cube tray)
- 1 tsp. torn fresh mint leaves + sprigs for garnishing
- 2 C. Greek yogurt
- 1 vanilla bean (split lengthwise)
- ½ C. honey
- ½ water

How it's made:

- In a saucepan over low heat, combine vanilla bean pod, honey, and water. Simmer for 7-9 min. to allow time for vanilla to infuse into honey. Remove vanilla bean pod and allow time for the mixture to cool completely.
- Combine some of the vanilla honey with yogurt, mint and ½ tray of coconut water in a blender. Blend until smooth in texture.
- Put mixture into glasses. Garnish with a sprig of mint. Serve cold!

Almond-Honey Power Bar

Preparation time: 30 min.

Complete time: 1 hour

Calories 246 – Carbs 38g – Sodium 57mg – Fat 10g

What's in it:

- 1/8 tsp. salt
- ¼ C. honey
- ½ tsp. vanilla extract
- ¼ C. turbinado sugar
- ¼ C. creamy almond butter
- 1/3 C. golden raisins
- 1/3 C. currants
- 1/3 C. dried apricots
- 1 C. unsweetened whole-grain puffed cereal
- 1 tbsp. sesame seeds
- 1 tbsp. flax seeds
- ¼ C. slivered almonds
- ¼ C. unsalted sunflower seeds
- 1 C. old-fashioned rolled oats

How it's made:

- Ensure oven is preheated to 350 degrees. With cooking spray, grease an 8" square pan.
- On a baking sheet with a rim, spread out sesame seeds, flaxseeds, sunflower seeds, almonds, and oats. Bake about 10 min. until oats are just toasted and nuts are fragrant. Pour in large bowl and add raisins, apricots, currants, and cereal. Toss to ensure thorough combination.
- In a small saucepan, mix together salt, vanilla, honey sugar and almond butter on low heat, ensuring to constantly stir. Perform this action 2 to 5 min. until mixture starts to bubble.
- Quickly pour almond butter batter into dry components, stirring to ensure there are no more visible lumps. Transfer to pan.
- Coat your hands with greasing medium of choice and press mixture into an even layer. Frost for 30 min. or until firm. Cut into 8 bars. Enjoy!

Orange Resolution Smoothie

Time: 5 min.

Calories 109 – Carbs 12g – Sodium 98mg – Fat 3g

What's in it:

- 1 banana
- ¼ C. honey
- 1 C. pineapple chunks
- 1 C. orange juice
- 1 C. mini carrots
- 2 C. Greek yogurt
- 2 C. frozen peach slices
- 2 C. frozen mango chunks

How it's made:

- Add all the above components into a blender.

- Blender on high until the consistency comes out creamy and smooth. Enjoy!

Creamy Kale and Eggs

Time: 25 min.

Calories 190 – Carbs 14g – Sodium 213mg – Fat 7g

What's in it:

- 4 slices of toasted crusty bread
- 2 tbsp. grated Parmesan
- 4 large eggs
- ¼ C. 2% Greek yogurt
- Pepper and salt
- Pinch of grated nutmeg
- 1 bunch of kale (stems remove and cut crosswise into thin ribbons)
- 2 tbsp. chopped leeks (both white and green parts)
- 1 tbsp. extra-virgin olive oil

How it's made:

- In a pan over intermediate to immense warmth, warm up oil. Pour in leeks and decrease warmth to low. Cook leeks 8 min. until softened but not browned.
- Pour in kale with leeks and cook 2 min. until wilted. Sprinkle with salt, pepper, and nutmeg to season. Then mix in yogurt. Combine well.
- Make four indentations in the kale and crack an egg into each one. Top each egg with pepper and salt to season.
- Top pan and cook 2 to 3 min. until egg whites are firm and eggs are cooked to the doneness you desire.
- Dive eggs and kale among 4 plates and top with parmesan cheese. Serve with crusty toasted bread.

Lunch Recipes

Grilled Sweet Potato and Scallion Salad

Preparation time: 10 min.

Complete time: 1 hour

Calories 151 – Carbs 5g – Sodium 4g – Fat 14g

What's in it:

- ¼ C. fresh, roughly cut up parsley
- Pepper and salt
- 1 tsp. honey
- 1 tbsp. balsamic vinegar
- 2 tbsp. apple cider vinegar
- 2 tbsp. Dijon mustard
- 2/3 C. extra-virgin olive oil
- 8 scallions
- 4 large sweet potatoes

How it's made:

- Ensure oven is preheated to 375 degrees. Bake potatoes for 45 min. until softened. Let cool a bit before cutting into large chunks.
- Preheat a grill on high heat. Brush sweet potatoes and scallions with 1/3 cup olive oil.
- Arrange them on grill and grill until they are tender, which takes around 5 min. Remove from grill and cut scallions into smaller pieces.
- Whisk remaining olive oil with mustard, honey, and

vinegar, seasoning with pepper and salt. Put in the potatoes, parsley, and scallions into this mixture and gently toss until everything is well coated.

Israeli Couscous Tabouli

Preparation time: 20 min.
Complete time: 28 min.

Calories 180 – Carbs 11g – Sodium 9.8g – Fat 13g

What's in it:

- 3 chopped scallions
- 2 ripe, seeded/diced tomatoes
- 2 tbsp. freshly chopped mint
- ½ C. freshly chopped cilantro
- 1 C. finely chopped parsley
- 3 tbsp. olive oil
- 1 zested and juiced lemon
- Pepper and salt
- 1 C. Israeli couscous

How it's made:

- Over intermediate warmth, pour water in a pot, sprinkle with salt and warm up to a boiling point.
- Pour in couscous and cook it until al dente, around 7 to 8 min. Remove liquid from couscous and set to the side to allow time to cool off a bit.
- Mix together olive oil and lemon juice/zest to create a vinaigrette. Sprinkle pepper and salt if needed to adequately season.
- Mix together scallions, tomatoes, mint, cilantro, parsley and couscous until combined. Toss everything with vinaigrette, seasoning with pepper and salt to achieve desired taste.
- Let the mixture to sit 30 min. so that their flavors can marry together before sitting down and consuming!

Frittata with Asparagus, Tomato, and Fontina

Preparation time: 15 min.
Complete time: 27 min.

Calories 230 – Carbs 11g – Sodium 9g – Fat 12g

What's in it:

- 3 ounces of diced Fontina
- Salt
- 1 seeded/diced tomato
- 12-ounces asparagus (trimmed/cut into ¼-1/2" pieces)
- 1 tbsp. butter
- 1 tbsp. olive oil
- ¼ tsp. pepper
- ½ tsp. salt
- 2 tbsp. whipping cream
- 6 large eggs

How it's made:

- Ensure that your broiler is preheated.
- Whisk together salt, pepper, cream, and eggs.
- In an ovenproof skillet, warm up butter on intermediate to immense warmth.
- Pour in asparagus, sautéing about 2 min. until pieces are crisp-tender.
- Raise heat to intermediate and add in the egg mixture onto asparagus, cooking for a bit to allow eggs to set.
- Top with cheese and decrease heat to medium or low, cooking frittata until set but the top is runny.
- Put the skillet into the broiler. Cook for 5 min. until the top of frittata is firmed and golden in color. Let stand 2 min. before removing from skillet.

Un-fried Chicken

Preparation time: 10 min.
Complete time: 55 min.

Calories 230 – Carbs 14g – Sodium 10g – Fat – 14g

What's in it:

- 1 ¼ C. cornflake crumbs
- Zest and juice from 1 lemon
- 2 egg whites
- ½ tsp. hot sauce
- ¼ C. low-fat buttermilk
- ½ tsp. chicken seasoning (recipe below)
- 8 skinless, boneless chicken thighs (visible fat trimmed off)
- Non-stick cooking spray

Chicken Seasoning:

- 1 C. salt
- ¼ C. garlic powder
- ¼ C. black pepper

How it's made:

- Ensure oven is preheated to 375 degrees. Grease a cast-iron pan with the greasing medium of your choice. Put over intermediate to immense warmth.
- Sprinkle thighs with chicken seasoning.
- Combine lemon juice/zest, egg whites, buttermilk and hot sauce in a large bowl until combined. Toss in chicken, coating thoroughly.

102

- Pour cornflake crumbs into another bowl. Dip chicken into these crumbs, pressing gently so that they adhere to chicken.
- Then place chicken in skillet and pop in the oven.
- Back forty to forty-five min. until chicken is golden and a device that reads meat temperature reads 165 degrees or higher.

Chicken and Rice Paprikash Casserole

Preparation time: 10 min.

Complete time: An hour and 50 min.

Calories 311 – Carbs 12g – Sodium 10g – Fat 15g

What's in it:

- 6 tbsp. decreased-fat sour cream
- 2 tbsp. chopped flat-leaf parsley
- 3 C. frozen brown rice (thawed)
- 2 C. low-sodium chicken broth
- 2 tbsp. tomato paste
- 1 tsp. hot paprika or ¼ tsp. cayenne pepper
- 1 tbsp. sweet Hungarian paprika
- 2 large finely chopped red bell peppers
- 2 onions, chopped
- 5 finely chopped cloves of garlic
- 1 tsp. extra virgin olive oil
- Pepper and salt
- 2 pounds of bone-in, skinless chicken thighs

How it's made:

- Ensure oven is preheated to 350 degrees. Pour chicken in a ceramic baking dish. Season with pepper and salt. Bake twenty-five to thirty min., until chicken is just cooked.
- While chicken is cooking, in a saucepan, warm up oil and add in salt, ¼ teaspoon salt, bell peppers, onions, and garlic. Cook 15 min., mixing around every once in a while until veggies are tender. If mixture becomes too dry, do not be afraid to add a tablespoon or two of water.

- Stir in sweet and hot paprika, cooking for 1 minute. Pour in tomato paste and cook for an additional minute.
- Put chicken broth and 2 cups of water into the pan. Rise up to boiling point, reducing warmth so that a nice simmer is maintained.
- Simmer mixture 5 min. until it becomes thickened.
- Put chicken on a plate and spread rice into the bottom of a dish meant to cook casseroles, topping with chicken and all the juices that it accumulated while cooking.
- Bake 40 min. until casserole is browned on the top.
- Top with parsley and serve alongside a nice dollop of sour cream if you so choose.

Tropical Chicken Patties

Preparation time: 15 min.

Complete time: 40 min.

Calories 517 – Carbs 56g – Sodium 219g – Fat 6g

What's in it:

- ¼ C. chopped fresh cilantro
- 1 ½ C. diced pineapple
- 1 C. frozen peas (thawed)
- 1 C. long grained white rice
- ¼ tsp. turmeric
- 1 finely chopped small red onion
- 2 ½ tbsp. vegetable oil
- Pepper and salt
- ½ tsp. ground allspice
- 2 minced cloves of garlic
- 2 small jalapeño peppers (1 green/1 red – seeded/diced)
- 1 ¼ pounds ground chicken

How it's made:

- In a large bowl, mix up chicken, half of the jalapeño, half the garlic, allspice, ¼ teaspoon salt and ¼ teaspoon pepper until combined.
- Then create four ½" patties. Put patties on a plate and placed covered in the fridge until you are ready to cook them.
- In a large skillet over medium heat, heat up 1 tablespoon vegetable oil. Pour in half the red onion, remaining jalapeño and garlic and turmeric. Cook for 1 minute.
- Add the rice, ¼ teaspoon salt and 2 cups of water. Bring

106

this to a boil.

- Decrease heat to medium-low. Cover and simmer for 15 min. until rice is tender. Add in the peas but cease to stir. Cover and set to the side.
- In a non-stick skillet over intermediate to immense warmth, heat up 1 tablespoon of oil. Add the patties to oil and cook for 4 min. on each side.
- Tin a bowl, toss pineapple cilantro, red jalapeño, remaining red onion and ½ tablespoon vegetable oil. Season with pepper and salt.
- Stir rice and peas and then season with pepper and salt to taste.
- Serve with patties and pineapple salsa.

Healthy Summer Pasta Salad

Preparation time: 25 min.
Complete time: 40 min.

Calories 207 – Carbs 11g – Sodium 11.4g – Fat 8g

What's in it:

- 1 zucchini (cut into small pieces)
- 1 ear of corn (husked and kernels cut from cob)
- 2 tbsp. chopped dill or fresh chives
- 1 C. cherry or grape tomatoes (halved and quartered)
- Pepper and salt, to taste
- ¾ tsp. dry mustard
- 1 ½ tsp. sugar
- 1 ½ tbsp. cider vinegar
- 3 tbsp. sour cream
- ½ C. mayo
- ¼ of one red onion (diced)
- 8 ounces dry cavatappi

How's it made:

- In a large pot, bring salted water to a boil. Add in cavatappi and cook it according to the package. Remove liquid and rinse in cold water. Set to the side.
- While cavatappi is cooking, soak onion in cold water for 5 min. and remove liquid.
- In a bowl, whisk together salt, pepper, remove liquidated red onion, mustard, sugar, oil, vinegar, sour cream and may until combined.
- Pour in zucchini, corn, dill, tomatoes and cooked cavatappi into the dressing. Stir well to coat everything thoroughly. Enjoy!

Chicken Peanut Stir-Fry

Preparation time: 15 min.
Complete time: 25 min.

Calories 476 – Carbs 48g – Sodium 315mg – Fat 14g

What's in it:

- ¼ C. roasted salted peanuts
- 1 small head of Napa cabbage (cored/cut into 2" pieces)
- 1 jalapeño pepper (seeded/thinly sliced)
- 1 bunch of scallions
- One 2" piece of ginger
- 2 tbsp. peanut or vegetable oil
- 1 pound skinless and boneless chicken breasts
- 1 tbsp + 1 tsp. rice vinegar
- 1 tbsp. + 2 tsp. cornstarch
- 3 tsp. soy sauce
- 1 C. basmati rice

How it's made:

- Cook rice according to directions.
- As rice cooks, whisk together 2 teaspoons soy cause and a tablespoon cornstarch and rice vinegar. Pour in chicken and thoroughly coat all sides.
- Mix together remaining cornstarch, 1/3 cup of water, brown sugar and 1 teaspoon soy sauce/rice vinegar in another bowl.
- In a large skillet over immense warmth, warm up a tablespoon of peanut oil. Pour in chicken and stir-fry 2 to 3 min. until lightly golden in color. Remove with slotted spoon to a bowl that is clean.

- Clean out the pan, return to high heat and pour in the peanut oil that remains. When it starts to smoke, add jalapeño, scallion whites, and ginger, stir-frying for 45 seconds to 1 minute. Add in cabbage, stir-frying for three to five min. just until crispy yet tender. Mix in brown sugar mixture and add with chicken. Stir-fry the sauce for 1-2 min. until it is thick and chicken is cooked all the way through.
- Mix in peanuts and scallion greens.
- Serve alongside rice.

Kale and Turkey Rice Bowl

Preparation time: 15 min.

Complete time: 40 min.

Calories 119 – Carbs 13g – Sodium 175mg – Fat 3g

What's in it:

- 2 ½ C. cooked white or brown rice
- One 5 oz. package of chopped kale (6 packed cups)
- ½ pound red skinned potatoes (cut into ½" pieces)
- 1 tsp. ground cumin
- 2 finely chopped cloves garlic
- 1 finely chopped onion
- 1 pound 93% lean ground turkey
- 1 tbsp. vegetable oil
- Salt
- 3 tbsp. sliced almonds
- 1 jalapeño pepper (halved and seeds removed)
- 1 bunch of cilantro (tough stems removed)

How it's made:

- In a blender, puree 3 tablespoons cilantro, ½ cup of water, jalapeño, almonds and ¼ teaspoon of salt until smooth in texture.
- In a large pot or Dutch oven over intermediate to immense warmth, heat vegetable oil. Add in turkey and ½ teaspoon of salt. Cook for 4 min., stirring to break up turkey with a wooden spoon. Cook until browned.
- Add cumin, garlic, and onion to meat, stirring occasionally until softened. Then pour in 1 ½ cups of water, pureed cilantro mixture, potatoes, and kale.

111

Cover and bring to a boil.
- Uncover and decrease heat to around medium. Let simmer for 15 min., stirring occasionally until potatoes are tender.
- Seasons with pepper and salt as desired. Serve over rice, garnished with leftover cilantro.

Escarole with Pancetta

Calories 124 – Carbs 5g – Sodium 224mg – Fat 2g

What's in it:

- 3 tbsp. diced pancetta
- 2 tbsp olive oil
- 4 garlic cloves
- 1 head chopped escarole

How it's made:

- Cool pancetta until crispy, remove liquid on a paper towel.
- In a skillet cook olive oil and smashed garlic cloves for 1 minute.
- Then add chopped escarole to the pan, cooking for 5 min. until wilted.
- Add pancetta to escarole in a serving dish and season with pepper.

Snack and Side Recipes

Roasted Sweet Potatoes with Honey and Cinnamon

Preparation time: 15 min.
Complete time: 45 min.

Calories 143 – Carbs 11g – Sodium 7g – Fat 23g

What's in it:

- Pepper and salt, to taste
- 2 tsp. ground cinnamon
- ¼ C. honey
- ¼ C. extra-virgin olive oil + more for drizzling onto cooked potatoes
- 4 sweet potatoes (peeled and cut into 1" cubes)

How it's made:

- Ensure oven is preheated to 375 degrees.
- In a roasting tray, lay out sweet potato cubes. Shower them in oil and honey and then top them with cinnamon, pepper, and salt.
- Roast 25 to 30 min. until tender.
- Pull out from the oven and pour onto a serving platter. Drizzle with additional olive oil before serving.

Garlic Mashed Cauliflower

Preparation time: 10 min.
Complete time: 20 min.

What's in it:

- Freshly chopped rosemary, for garnish
- Freshly ground black pepper
- 1 smashed and chopped small clove of garlic
- 1 tbsp. non-fat Greek yogurt
- 1 tbsp. extra-virgin olive oil
- 2 tbsp. grated Parmesan cheese
- ¼ C. chicken stock
- Salt
- 1 medium head of cauliflower, chopped

How it's made:

- In a big pot, raise water up to the point of boiling. Pour in chopped cauliflower and salt. Cook cauliflower 10 min. until it's tenderized.
- Allow time to remove liquid and then dry with a paper towel.
- In a food processor, pour in hot cauliflower with chicken stock, garlic, yogurt, olive oil, and cheese. Process components until they are smooth in texture.
- Stir in a dash of pepper and salt if needed. Proceed in adding in chopped rosemary.
  Serve!

Strawberry Oatmeal Bars

Preparation time: 10 min.
Complete time: An hour and 20 min.

Calories 136 – Carbs 18g – Sodium 9g – Fat 8.9g

What's in it:

- 1 10-12-ounce jar of strawberry preserves
- ½ tsp. salt
- 1 tsp. baking powder
- 1 C. packed brown sugar
- 1 ½ C. rolled oats
- 1 ½ C. regular white baking flour
- 1 ¾ sticks of unsalted butter (cut into pieces)

How it's made:

- Ensure oven is preheated to 350 degrees. Butter up a rectangular pan.
- Mix salt, baking powder, brown sugar, oat, flour, and butter together until combined.
- Press half of the oat mixture into pan. Then lay out the strawberry preserves over it.
- Top the other half of oat mixture over preserve layer and pat down gently.
- Bake 30 to 40 min. until light brown in color.
- Let cool completely before cutting them into squares.

Fresh Corn Salad

Preparation time: 10 min.

Complete time: 13 min.

Calories 134 – Carbs 6g – Sodium 3g – Fat 9g

What's in it:

- ½ C. julienned fresh basil leaves
- ½ tsp. black pepper
- ½ tsp. salt
- 3 tbsp. olive oil
- 3 tbsp. cider vinegar
- ½ C. small-diced red onion
- 5 ears of shucked corn

How it's made:

- Warm a salted pot of water up to a boil over immense warmth, cooking up corn for 3 min. to decrease starchiness. Remove liquid. Then pour into ice water to stop cooking in order to set the bright, yellow color.
- Once corn is cooled, cut kernels from the cob.
- Pour kernels into onions, salt, pepper, vinegar, and oil of olive in a big bowl. Before eating, mix with fresh basil. Sprinkle with seasonings of choice until you reach desired taste.
- Serve at room temperature or cold.

Kale Chips

Preparation time: 10 min.
Complete time: 1 hour and 25 min.

Calories 17 – Carbs 1g – Sodium .9g – Fat 0g

What's in it:

- Salt
- 1 tsp. za'atar spice
- 1 tsp. dried Mexican oregano
- Olive oil
- 10 kale leaves (washed, dried, stems discarded)

How it's made:

- Ensure oven is preheated to 225 degrees.
- Pour leaves of kale into a bowl and lightly put olive oil over kale until leaves are thoroughly coated and glistening.
- Sprinkle oregano and za'atar over the top of kale. Season with salt and toss gently.
- Transfer kale to baking sheet. Back 45 min. – 1 hour until crispy. Let cool before serving.

Pomegranate Quinoa Pilaf

Preparation time: 15 min.
Complete time: 45 min.

Calories 248 – Carbs 27g – Sodium 89mg - Fat 1g

What's in it:

- ½ C. toasted slivered almonds
- Pepper and salt
- 1 tsp. sugar
- 1 tsp. fresh lemon zest
- ½ a lemon's juice
- 1 tbsp. flat leaf parsley, chopped
- ½ C. scallions (diagonally sliced)
- ½ C. pomegranate seeds
- 2 C. low-sodium chicken broth
- 1 C. quinoa
- ½ medium onion (diced)
- 2 tbsp. olive oil

How it's made:

- In a pan over intermediate to immense warmth, warm up a tablespoon of oil. Sauté the onion until translucent in color and fragrant. Pour in your quinoa and mix to ensure an even coating.
- Add chicken broth and warm up over immense warmth until it reaches the point of boiling. Decrease warmth and simmer twenty min. until liquid is quinoa soaks up liquid and is nice and tender.
- Mix together sugar, lemon juice, lemon zest, parsley, scallions, pomegranate seeds and oil until combined.

Pour in quinoa and sprinkle with pepper and salt to season until you reach desired taste.

- Garnish with toasted slivered almonds.

Healthy Cauliflower Rice

Preparation time: 10 min.
Complete time: 25 min.

Calories 189 – Carbs 14g – Sodium 27g – Fat 2g

What's in it:

- Juice of ½ lemon
- 2 tbsp. finely chopped parsley leaves
- Salt
- 1 finely diced medium onion
- 3 tbsp. olive oil
- A head of cauliflower

How it's made:

- Trim cauliflower florets, cutting as much of the stem off as possible. Break up florets and pulse in 3 batches in a food processor until mixture is similar to couscous.
- Within a pan over intermediate to immense warmth, warm up oil. As the oil just begins to smoke a bit, add onions, stirring to coat. Cooking onions for 8 min., stirring constantly, until they are golden brown on the edges and soft in texture.
- Add cauliflower, combining well. Then add 1 teaspoon of salt and cook 3 to 5 min. until cauliflower is tender. Take way from the heat.
- In a large serving bowl pour in cauliflower. Garnish with parsley, lemon juice and pepper and salt. Serve warm!

Vanilla Almonds

Preparation time: 5 min.
Complete time: 55 min.

Calories 25 – Carbs 12g – Sodium 12g – Fat 9g

What's in it:

- ½ tsp. ground cinnamon
- ¼ tsp. salt
- ¾ C. sugar
- 4 C. whole almonds
- 1 tsp. pure vanilla extract
- 1 beaten egg white

How it's made:

- Ensure oven is preheated to 300 degrees.
- Mix egg white with vanilla extract, then pour in almonds and stir to ensure even coatings.
- Combine cinnamon, salt, and sugar. Then add to egg white mixture, stirring together well.
- Pour mixture into solitary layer onto a sheet meant for baking that has been liberally greased.
- Bake 20 min.
- Take out of the oven and let cool on waxed paper and then tear into clusters.

Watermelon and Cucumber Smoothie

Time: 5 min.

Calories 98 – Carbs 10g – Sodium 3g – Fat 0.5g

What's in it:

- 2 C. cubed seedless watermelon (frozen)
- Juice of half a lime (1 tbsp.)
- 1 tbsp. honey (optional)
- 3 tbsp. low-fat buttermilk
- One 2" piece English cucumber (peeled/chopped)

How it's made:

- In a blender, blend honey, lime juice, buttermilk, and cucumber on high until smooth in texture.
- Add half of the frozen watermelon and blend until smooth and well combined. Push down components with a soon before adding in remaining watermelon. Blend until entirety of mix is smooth. Add 1 to 2 tablespoons water if you need to so that you are able to get the right consistency.
- Put into a glass garnished with a cucumber slice.

Slow Cooker Spiced Nuts

Preparation time: 5 min.
Complete time: 4 hours and 5 min.

Calories 89 – Carbs 9g – Sodium 349mg – Fat 9g

What's in it:

- 2 C. unsalted roasted cashews
- 2 C. raw pecans
- 1/8 tsp. cayenne pepper
- 1 tsp. salt
- 2 tsp. orange zest
- 2 tsp. cinnamon
- 3 tbsp. melted unsalted butter
- ¼ C. pure maple syrup

How it's made:

- Line a 6-quart slow cooker with heavy duty foil and liberally grease with greasing medium of choice. Set aside.
- Mix together cayenne, salt, orange zest, cinnamon, butter and maple syrup. Add nuts to the bowl and toss gently to coat thoroughly.
- Pour nuts into the slow cooker in a nice even layer, cover and turn to high.
- Cook for an hour until light syrup forms at the bottom.
- Decrease the warmth to low, stir nuts and cook for another hour, mixing up about every 20 min.
- Turn slow cooker off, uncover and let nuts harder for 2 hours, stirring occasionally.
- Nuts can be stored for 5 days if you do not enjoy right away.

Spicy Summer Squash with Herbs

Preparation time: 10 min.

Complete time: 25 min.

Calories 101 – Carbs 12g – Sodium 201mg – Fat 5g

What's in it:

- ¼ C. minced fresh chives
- 1 minced clove of garlic
- 2 tsp. finely chopped fresh sage or rosemary
- Pepper and salt
- 1 ½ tsp. white wine vinegar
- 1 diced onion
- 1 minced small jalapeño (leave some seeds within)
- 3 medium yellow or green summer squash (diced)
- 1 ½ tbsp. extra-virgin olive oil

How it's made:

- Within a pan on intermediate to immense warmth, warm up oil. Pour in pepper and salt, vinegar, onions, jalapeños, and squash, stirring to combine. Cover and cook 6 min. until squash starts to become brown in color.
- Remove lid and continue cooking process for another 6 min. until squash is browned nicely. Add sage and garlic and cook for another minute. Sprinkle with pepper and salt to season in order to achieve desired taste.
- Stir in chives. Pour into a bowl and serve!

Pumpkin-Parmesan Biscuits

Preparation time: 30 min.
Complete time: 50 min.

Calories 105 – Carbs 12g – Sodium 200mg – Fat 5g

What's in it:

- ¼ C. heavy cream
- ½ C. canned pure pumpkin
- 1 stick cold unsalted butter + more for brushing (diced)
- 2 tbsp. finely grated parmesan cheese
- ¼ tsp. freshly grated nutmeg
- 1 tsp. salt
- 1 tbsp. sugar
- 1 tbsp. baking powder
- 2 C. all-purpose flour + more for dusting

How it's made:

- Ensure oven is preheated to 400 degrees. With parchment paper, line a sheet in which you can bake on.
- Mix nutmeg, salt, sugar baking powder, and flour together. Then add in 1 tablespoon of parmesan. Add in diced butter and with the mixture with fingertips until it resembles coarse crumbs.
- In a separate bowl, mix cream and pumpkin together and put over flour mixture. Mix with hands or a fork to create a softened dough.
- Put dough on a flat surface that has been mildly floured. Roll out into ¾" thick rectangle using a floured rolling pin.
- Cut out biscuits and arrange them on the baking sheet

about 2" apart. Pour a bit of nicely melted butter over the tops before sprinkling with remaining parmesan.

- Bake 15 - 20 min. until biscuits are richly colored.
- Let sit on a rack made of wire to cool. Allow cooling a bit before serving.

Potatoes with Chili Butter

Preparation time: 5 min.
Complete time: 25 min.

Calories 165 – Carbs 20g – Sodium 174mg – Fat 9g

What's in it:

- 1 pound of new potatoes
- ½ tsp. chili powder
- 3 tbsp. butter
- Pepper and salt

How it's made:

- In a pot of cold salted water, add one pound of new potatoes. Warm up to the point of boiling and cook fifteen to twenty min. until potatoes become tenderized. Remove liquid them.
- In a pan, melt 3 tablespoons of butter and add ½ teaspoon of chili powder as well as a sprinkle or two of pepper and salt to season.
- Drizzle chili butter over potatoes. A great side!

Tomato Gratin

Preparation time: 4 min.
Complete time: 15 min.

Calories 109 – Carbs 12g – Sodium 123mg – Fat 2g

What's in it:

- 2 pints of grape tomatoes
- 4 garlic cloves
- ¼ C. olive oil
- 2 tsp. fresh thyme
- ½ C. parmesan
- ½ C. breadcrumbs

How it's made:

- In an ovenproof skillet over intermediate to immense warmth, cook grape tomatoes, smash garlic cloves, ¼ cup of olive oil and thyme for 8 min. until tomatoes are softened.
- Within the means of a bowl, mix remaining olive oil, breadcrumbs, and parmesan together.
- Sprinkle parmesan mixture over tomatoes.
- Broil 3 min. until the dish is a golden brown color.

Eggplant Caponata

Complete Time: 25 min.

Calories 138 – Carbs 14g – Sodium 199mg – Fat 1g

What's in it:

- 1 chopped onion
- ¼ C. olive oil
- 1 stalk of celery, chopped
- 1 eggplant, chopped
- 1 chopped red bell pepper
- 3 tbsp. golden raisins
- 1 tbsp. chopped oregano
- ½ C. water
- 1 C. halved grape tomatoes
- 1 tbsp. cider vinegar
- 1 tbsp. capers
- Pepper and salt, to taste
- Torn basil, for garnish

How it's made:

- In a pan, cook onion alongside olive oil 3 min. Then pour in celery and eggplant and cook an additional 4 min.
- Pour in red bell pepper, cooking for 3 min. Then pour in raisins, oregano, and water. Bubble for eight min.
- Pour in capers, apple cider vinegar, and grape tomatoes. Cook for 7 min.
- Sprinkle with pepper and salt to season in order to achieve desired taste and garnish with basil before serving.

Italian Lentil Salad

Preparation time: 8 min.

Complete time: 28 min.

Calories 198 – Carbs 11g – Sodium 89mg – Fat 2g

What's in it:

Salad:

- 2 tsp. lemon zest
- ½ C. coarsely chopped skinned/toasted hazelnuts
- 1 red bell pepper that has been seeded and diced
- 1 cucumber that has been peeled, seeded and diced
- 1 C. seedless red grapes that have been cut in half
- 1 C. seedless green grapes that have been cut in half
- 2 scallions, cut up
- 1 pound green lentils (Sabarot recommended)

Vinaigrette:

- ¼ tsp. ground black pepper
- ½ tsp. salt
- 1/3 C. extra-virgin olive oil
- 1/3 C. fresh lemon juice

How it's made:

- *For the salad:* Get out a pot. Pour in water and salt and warm up liquid up to the point of boiling. Pour in lentils and cook 18 - 20 min. until tenderized, ensuring to stir periodically. Remove liquid. Let cool off for 5 min. at the very least.

- Pour lentils and remaining salad components into a large salad bowl.
- *For vinaigrette:* In a small bowl, pour in lemon juice. Gradually add in oil, mixing rapidly until incorporated. Sprinkle with pepper and salt to season in order to achieve desired taste. Enjoy!

Dinner Recipes

Oven Baked Salmon

Preparation time: 5 min.
Complete time: 20 min.

Calories 290 – Carbs 17g – Sodium 11g – Fat 9g

What's in it:

- 12-ounce salmon fillet
- Coarse salt
- Black pepper
- Toasted almond parsley salad (for serving)
- Baked squash (optional: for serving)

Toasted Almond Parsley Salad

- Extra-virgin olive oil
- ½ C. toasted almonds
- 1 C. flat-leaf parsley
- 2 tbsp. rinsed capers
- Coarse salt
- 1 tbsp. red wine vinegar
- 1 shallot

How it's made:

- Ensure oven is preheated to 450 degrees.
- Sprinkle fillets of salmon with pepper and salt to season.
- Put salmon on a baking sheet, with the skin side touching the pan, preferably non-stick.
- Bake twelve to fifteen min. until salmon is cooked all the

way through.
- Serve with toasted almond parsley salad if you desire!

Toasted Almond Parsley Salad:

- Slice and dice shallot then pour vinegar over shallots, adding a pinch of salt to season. Allow time for the mixture to sit for 30 min.
- Cut up almonds, capers, and parsley, adding to shallots. Pour in olive oil to taste. Mix and adjust seasonings as needed.

Pork Tenderloin with Seasoned Rub

Preparation time: 5 min.
Complete time: 35 min.

Calories 310 – Carbs 29g – Sodium 10g – Fat 18g

What's in it:

- 1 tsp. minced garlic
- 1 tbsp. olive oil
- 1 ¼ pounds of pork tenderloin
- Salt, to taste
- 1 tsp. dried thyme
- 1 tsp. ground coriander
- 1 tsp. ground cumin
- 1 tsp. dried oregano
- 1 tsp. garlic powder

How it's made:

- Ensure oven is preheated to 450 degrees.
- Mix all dry components until well incorporated. This is the rub for your tenderloin.
- Sprinkle rub over tenderloin and proceed to rub into all sides of meat.
- Pour olive oil in a pan over intermediate to immense warmth. Pour in garlic and proceed to sauté for a minute, stirring constantly.
- Place tenderloin in the pan, cooking 10 min. per side, turning meat with tongs.
- Upon a nice roasting pan, place your meat and bake 20 min.
- Cut, serve and enjoy!

Mushroom Stuffer Pork Tenderloin

Preparation Time: 25 min.

Complete time: 1 hour and 10 min.

Calories 290 – Carbs 12g – Sodium 13g – Fat 23g

What's in it:

- ½ tsp. grated lemon zest
- 2 pork tenderloins
- ½ C. chopped fresh parsley
- 1 tbsp. breadcrumbs
- 1 clove of garlic
- Pepper and salt
- 8 ounces of thinly sliced cremini mushrooms
- 4 slices chopped low-sodium bacon
- 5 tbsp. extra virgin olive oil + extra for basting

How it's made:

- In a large pan over intermediate to immense warmth, warm up 2 tablespoons of oil. Pour in bacon and cook about eight min. until nice and crispy.
- Pour in mushrooms, ½ tsp. pepper and salt and cook mushrooms until soft.
- Pour in garlic and cook for a minute.
- Take pan away from heat and mix in breadcrumbs and all but a couple tablespoons of parsley until combined. Set aside to cool.
- Immerse ten to twelve toothpicks in liquid to avoid burning them in the oven later. Rinse off meat and then dry graciously. Butterfly cut the tenderloin, cutting it like a book so that meat ends up lying flat.

- Cover pork in a wrap made of plastic and beat with a meat hammer until it is ½" thick.
- Spread mushroom mixture over tenderloins and secure the seams with soaked toothpicks.
- Preheat grill on intermediate to immense warmth, brushing the grates with olive oil. Brush pork rolls with oil and season with pepper and salt.
- Grill tenderloins, turning frequently until a thermometer says 140 degrees. Transfer to a cutting board and let rest for 10 min.
- Mix up remaining olive oil and parsley with lemon zest, pepper, and salt. Remove toothpicks from meat and slice pork rolls. Top with parsley oil and serve.

Four-Step Lemon-Onion Chicken

Preparation time: 15 min.
Complete time: 40 min.

Calories 467 –Carbs 16g – Sodium 282mg – Fat 6g

What's in it:

- 4 boneless, skinless chicken breast halves (sliced in half horizontally)
- 1 9-ounce bag spinach
- Juice of 2 lemons
- 1 C. low-sodium chicken broth
- ¼ C. white wine (optional)
- 1 small bunch of fresh thyme leaves (chopped)
- 1 thinly sliced red onion
- ¼ C. all-purpose flour
- 3 tbsp. extra-virgin olive oil
- Pepper and salt, to taste
- 1 tsp. dried thyme

How it's made:

- Season chicken with thyme, pepper, and salt.
- In a large sauté pan over intermediate to immense warmth, heat olive oil.
- Put flour in a shallow dish and dredge chicken in batches.
- Adding chicken to pan, sauté on both sides for 3 min. per side. Transfer to plate and cover with foil.
- Add red onion and thyme to the pan and cook over low heat for 5 min., stirring every now and again until aromatic.

- Combine wine, chicken broth and lemon juice in a bowl. Turn heat up to high and deglaze broth mixture, scraping the pan with wooden spoon.
- Cook for about 10 min. until liquid starts to decrease. Remove from heat and whisk in 1 ½ tablespoons butter. Season with pepper and salt.
- Put spinach in a microwave-safe bowl and add 3 tablespoons water, covering loosely with plastic wrap. Microwave 5-6 min. until wilted.
- Remove liquid and toss with remaining butter, juice of other lemon and salt/pepper to taste.
- Arrange on serving platter on top of chicken. Spoon sauce over the top and serve!

Dry Rubbed London Broil

Preparation time: 8 min.
Complete time: 23 min.
Calories 219 – Carbs 12g – Sodium 110mg – Fat 11.8g

What's in it:

- 2 tbsp. olive oil
- One 2 pound London broil
- 1 recipe Dave's Rub

Dave's Rub
- 15 grinds black pepper
- 4 pinches salt
- 2 tsp. garlic powder
- 1 tbsp. sweet paprika
- 1 tbsp. dried oregano
- 2 tbsp. chili powder

How it's made:

- Rub London broil with olive oil and generously apply dry rub. Let sit for 15 min. at room temperature.
- Preheat a grill pan on intermediate to immense warmth.
- Place meat on grill and grill for 5 min. per side for medium-rare.
- Remove from heat and let rest for 5-10 min. before slicing.

Herbed Tuna Steaks

Preparation time: 1 hour and 10 min.
Complete time: 1 hour and 20 min.

Calories 198 – Carbs 12g – Sodium 209mg – Fat 9g

What's in it:

- Pepper and salt, to taste
- Two 1-pound center-cut tuna steaks (1" in thickness)
- 3 tbsp. extra-virgin olive oil
- 3 scallions
- 6 sprigs thyme (leaves stripped)
- 3 sprigs rosemary (leaves stripped)

How it's made:

- Roughly chop scallions, thyme, and rosemary and put into a small bowl, mix with a tablespoon of oil.
- Within a shallow dish, season tuna steaks with pepper and salt. Rub with herb mixture on both sides. Cover and Frost for 1-4 hours.
- In a pan on high heat, warm up remaining olive oil. Place tuna in skillet and sear two to three min. on each side until rich in color to achieve medium rare tuna steaks.
- Place on a board meant for cutting for 5 min. to rest before proceeding to slice. Enjoy!

Steamed Shrimp Dumplings

Preparation time: 1 hour
Complete time: 1 hour 40 min.

Calories 234 – Carbs 17g – Sodium 125mg – Fat 6g

What's in it:

- 36 round dumpling wrappers
- Pinch of white pepper
- ½ tsp. sugar
- Salt
- ¾ tsp. toasted sesame oil
- 1 ½ tsp. dry sherry
- 1 ½ tbsp. cornstarch
- 2 finely chopped scallions
- 1/3 C. water chestnuts, cut up finely
- ¾ pound large shrimp (peeled/deveined/chopped finely)
- 1 large egg white

Ponzu dipping sauce:

- 3 tbsp. ponzu sauce
- 1 tsp. soy sauce
- ½ tsp. sesame oil
- 1 chopped scallion

How it's made:

- In a large bowl, beat egg white. Add ¼ teaspoon salt, pepper, sugar, sesame oil, sherry, cornstarch, scallions, chestnuts, and shrimp. Combine well for 1 minute until it starts to thicken. Frost for 1 hour.

- On a clean surface covered with a damp paper towel, set out 1 dumpling wrapper. Stir 1 heaping teaspoon of shrimp mixture into the wrapper. Dab a finger into a bowl of cold water to moisten edges of the wrapper. Fold in half and press together the edges to seal. Place onto a sheet meant for baking. Perform this process with the remainder of dumpling wrappers.
- Fill up a pan with ¼" of water and bring to a boil. Working in batches, add dumplings in a single layer, cover and steam for 5 min. to cook.
- Transfer cooked dumpling to a plate.
- To make dipping sauce: mix all sauce components together in a small bowl until combined. Serve along with dumplings!

Braised Chicken with Mushrooms

Preparation time: 20 min.
Complete time: 3 hours and 10 min.

Calories 218 – Carbs 23g – Sodium 319mg – Fat 8g

What's in it:

- ½ C. celery tops or flat-leaf parsley (chopped)
- ½ - ¾ C. white wine
- 2 large bay leaves
- Few sprigs of thyme (finely chopped)
- 5-6 cloves of garlic (thinly sliced)
- 2 ribs celery (finely chopped)
- 2 carrots (finely chopped)
- 2 onions (sliced)
- 1 pound cremini mushrooms (thinly sliced)
- Pepper and salt, to taste
- 4 pieces of chicken leg quarters (Bone-in, skin on)
- Olive oil, for frying
- 2 C. chicken stock
- 1 ounce dried porcini mushrooms

How it's made:

- In a small pot over intermediate to immense warmth, pour in dried mushrooms and stock. Bring to boil and then decrease to low in order to reconstitute.
- In a large skillet with a lid, heat a thin layer of olive oil over intermediate to immense warmth. Pat chicken dry and season liberally with pepper and salt. Brown only half the chicken at a time, skin side down for 5 min. Then turn chicken and cook an additional 3-4 min. on another side.
- Remove browned chicken to a plate and place fresh mushrooms, cooking 10-15 min. Pour in salt, pepper, bay leaves, thyme, garlic, celery, carrot, and onion, stirring and cooking for another 10 min. until softened.
- Deglaze pot with white wine. Add chicken back into the pot and arrange veggies and mushrooms around it. Pour stock over chicken, reserving a few spoonfuls.
- Cover and braise on low, simmering for 30 min. Serve.

Coffee Rubbed Steak with Peppers and Onions

Preparation time: 30 min.
Complete time: 45 min.

Calories 321 – Carbs 23g – Sodium 334mg – Fat 9.8g

What's in it:

- Juice of ½ a lime + lime wedges for garnish
- 1 green bell pepper (cut into strips)
- Ground black pepper
- 1 onion (cut into wedges)
- 2 tsp. vegetable oil
- One 1 ¼ - 1 ½ inch skirt steak (cut into 4 pieces)
- Salt
- 1/8 tsp. ground cinnamon
- ½ tsp. ancho chili powder
- 1 tsp. mustard powder
- 1 tsp. unsweetened cocoa powder
- 1 tbsp. instant coffee
- 2 tbsp. + 1 tsp. pack light or dark brown sugar

How it's made:

- In a bowl, mix together 1 teaspoon salt, cinnamon, chili powder, mustard powder, cocoa powder, instant coffee and 2 tablespoons brown sugar. Rub between fingers until fine in texture.
  Season steak with salt and generously rub coffee-spice mixture on.
- In a cast-iron skillet over medium heat, heat up vegetable oil. Sear steak 3-6 min. on each side for medium rare. Put onto a cutting board and let rest. Reserve juices from the steak that are in skillet.
- Add remaining brown sugar and onion into the skillet, sprinkling with pepper and salt to taste. Cook on intermediate to immense warmth for 5 min. until onion is golden and soft.
- Then add bell pepper and ¼ cup of water, cooking for 5 min., stirring until crisp yet tender. Stir in lime juice, season with more pepper and salt.
- Slice skirt steak against the grain. Divide bell peppers, onions, and juices from steak among plates. Serve with lime wedges and cornbread.

Dessert Recipes

Angel Food Cake

Preparation time: 20 min.
Complete time: 55 min.

Calories 267 – Carbs 12g – Sodium 7g – Fat 13g

What's in it:

- 1 ½ tsp. cream of tartar
- 1 tsp. orange extract
- 1/3 C. warm water
- 12 egg whites (room temperature)
- 1 C. sifted cake flour
- ¼ tsp. salt
- 1 ¾ C. sugar

How it's made:

- Ensure oven is preheated to 350 degrees.
- Spin sugar in a food processor for 2 min. until sugar is super fine in texture.
- Sift half of sugar with salt and cake flour, setting another half aside.
- Whisk cream of tartar, orange extract, water and egg whites in a large bowl. Once you have whisked for 2 min., switch to a hand mixer.
- Slowly sift in reserved sugar, beating constantly at medium speed.
- When you have achieved medium peaks, sift enough of the flour mixture to dust the top of the foam. Using a

spatula, fold gently. Continue to do this until all of the flour mixtures is well incorporated.

- Spoon mixture carefully into an un-greased tube or bundt pan.
- Bake for 35 min. and check for doneness with a wooden skewer.
- Cool upside down on a cooling rack for at least 1 hour before attempting to remove from pan.

Cocoa Brownies

Preparation time: 15 min.
Complete time: 1 hour and 15 min.

Calories 200 – Carbs 11g – Sodium 4g – Fat 8g

What's in it:

- ½ tsp. salt
- ½ C. sifted flour
- 2 tsp. vanilla extract
- 1 ¼ C. sifted cocoa
- 8 ounces melted butter
- 1 C. sifted brown sugar
- 1 C. sifted sugar
- 4 eggs
- Flour, to dust pan
- Soft butter, for greasing pan

How it's made:

- Ensure oven is preheated to 300 degrees.
- Butter and flour an 8" square pan.
- Mix eggs until fluffy and light yellow in color. Then pour in both sugars and remaining components, mixing well until incorporated.
- Put batter into greased pan meant for baking. Bake 45 min. or until toothpick turns out with no more batter on it that has been inserted in the center.
- Once baked, set on a wire rack to allow to adequately cool.

Lemon Ricotta Cookies with Lemon Glaze

Preparation time: 15 min.

Complete time: 2 hours and 50 min.

Calories 149 – Carbs 9g – Sodium 4g – Fat 12g

What's in it:

- 1 zested lemon
- 3 tbsp. lemon juice
- 1 15 oz. container of whole milk ricotta cheese
- 2 eggs
- 2 C. sugar
- 1 stick softened unsalted butter
- 1 tsp. salt
- 1 tsp. baking powder
- 2 ½ C. regular white baking flour

Glaze:

- 1 zested lemon
- 3 tbsp. lemon juice
- 1 ½ C. powdered sugar

How it's made:

- Ensure oven is preheated to 375 degrees.
- Mary together salt, flour, and baking powder.
- In yet another bowl, cream up sugar and butter. With the help of a mixer that you plug in, combine butter and sugar for three min. until it is fluffy and very lightened in texture. Pour in eggs one at a time, mixing each you're your reach ensured blending. Then pour in ricotta

cheese, lemon zest/juice. Beat until combined.

- Mix in dry components.
- Line a couple of baking sheets with parchment paper. Pour cookie dough (2 tbsp. per cookie) onto sheets.
- Bake 15 min. until the edges of the cookies are slightly golden brown.
  Let cookies rest for 20 min.
- *For glaze:* Stir together lemon zest/juice and powdered sugar until smooth in texture. Spoon ½ teaspoon of glaze onto each cookie using the back of a spoon.
- Allow time for glaze harden (2 hours should be good!) Enjoy!

Espresso Chip Meringues

Calories 23 – Carbs 2g – Sodium .5g – Fat .5g

What's in it:

- 2/3 C. mini semi-sweet chocolate chips
- 2 tsp. instant espresso powder
- ¼ tsp. pure vanilla extract
- 1/8 tsp. cream of tartar
- ¾ C. superfine sugar
- Pinch of fine sea salt
- 3 larger egg whites (room temperature)

How it's made:

- Ensure oven is preheated to 300 degrees. Make sure that the rack that lives within the means of your oven is positioned in the center of your oven before preheating.
- With parchment paper, line a sheet and set to the side.
- Beat egg whites at low speed for a minute until fluffy. A tablespoon at a time, stir in your sugar. Then pour in cream of tartar, vanilla extract, and espresso powder.
- With the help of an electric mixer, beat mixture 3 to 5 min. until it is thick and holds stiff peaks. Fold in chocolate chips.
- Drop ¼-1/2 cupfuls of mixture onto baking sheet, ensuring there are at least 2 inches between each.
- Bake 30 min. Take out of the oven, rotating pan and pop back in the oven to bake another 30 min.
- Turn off oven, allowing meringues to sit in the oven to cool. This should take about 2 hours.
- Take out of the oven and allow time for them to cool down. You can store uneaten ones for up to 4 days in a container that seals well.

Healthy No-Bake Chocolate Peanut Butter Bars

Preparation time: 10 min.
Complete time: 4 hours and 10 min.

Calories 189 – Carbs 12g – Sodium 109mg – Fat 10g

What's in it:

Crust:
- 4 oz. melted semi-sweet chocolate morsels
- 3 tbsp. melted unsalted butter
- 24 chocolate wafer cookies
- Cooking spray

Filling:
- 2/3 C. confectioners' sugar
- ½ C. 2% Greek yogurt
- ½ C. creamy all-natural peanut butter
- 4 oz. decreased-fat cream cheese

Topping:
- Salt
- ¼ C. chopped unsalted peanuts

How it's made:

- *For crust:* Line an 8" square pan with foil, letting some hang over the side. Lightly coat with cooking spray.
- Process cookies until they are finely ground within the means of a food processor. Pour in melted butter during this process until crumbs are thoroughly coated with butter.

- Add in melted chocolate morsels and process until mixture resembles a wet sand texture.
- Press cookie mixture into bottom of the prepared pan. Cover and frost when filled. Clean out the food processor.
- *For the filling:* In the cleaned out processor pour in sugar, yogurt, peanut butter, and cream cheese, mixing until creamy and smooth.
- Pour mixture over cookie crust. Top with peanuts and sprinkle with ¼ teaspoon salt.
- Top with a cover and Frost within the means of your refrigerator for at least 4 hours or during the course of the night. Knife into twelve bars and serve!

Greek Yogurt Cheesecake

Preparation time: 20 min.

Complete time: 4 hours and 40 min.

Calories 211 – Carbs 21.1g – Sodium 132mg – Fat 12g

What's in it:

- 1 tsp. unflavored gelatin
- ¾ C. unsweetened pineapple juice
- 2 C. frozen wild blueberries
- Salt
- 1 tsp. lemon zest
- 1 tsp. vanilla extract
- ¼ C. all-purpose flour
- ¾ C. sugar
- 3 large eggs
- 8 ounces decreased-fat cream cheese (room temperature)
- One 17 oz. container of 2% Greek yogurt
- 2 tbsp. melted unsalted butter
- 2 C. slightly crushed cinnamon sugar pita chips

How it's made:

- Ensure oven is preheated to 325 degrees with the oven rack positioned in the center. Coat a 9" springform pan with greasing medium of your choice. Wrap sides and bottom of the pan with foil. Place pan on baking sheet.
- In a food processor, pulse pita chips until they are fine. Pour in butter and process until crumbs become moistened.
- Take the crumbs and press into the bottom of the pan, using about ½ of a cup along the sides.
- Bake crust for 5 min. until it looks slightly dry and fragrant.
- In a clean food processor, combine ½ teaspoon salt, lemon zest, vanilla, flour, sugar, eggs, cream cheese and yogurt until all components are smooth and well mixed.
- Add cream cheese mixture to the crust you prepared earlier.
- Bake 40 to 50 min. until middle is set.
- Allow time for the cheesecake to completely.
- Top with a cover and allow to Frost for at least 3 hours or during the course of the night.
- *For topping*: In a saucepan, bring blueberries and pineapple juice to the point of boiling. Decrease the warmth to low and simmer five min. Take away from the heat.
- Pour gelatin and 1 tablespoon of water into a bowl and allow to sit for 5 min. Then proceed to stir dissolved gelatin into hot berry mixture until well mixed. Put this mixture in another bowl and let Frost for at least 3 hours until thickened.
- Once cheesecake is Frosted, take away from the pan. Slice and consume with blueberry sauce topped over the top of the cake.

Apple and Berry Brown Betty

Preparation time: 25 min.
Complete time: 1 hour and 10 min.

Calories 290 – Carbs 17g – Sodium 390mg – Fat 11g

What's in it:

- Vanilla ice cream or whipped cream (optional topping)
- ½ tsp. salt
- ½ C. chopped almonds
- ½ C. packed light brown sugar
- 1 C. crushed sugar cones (about 6)
- 2 tbsp. all-purpose flour
- Zest and juice from ½ a lemon
- ½ tsp. nutmeg
- 1 tsp. cinnamon
- 1/3 C. granulated sugar
- 2 C. blackberries
- 4 Golden Delicious Apples
- 1 melted stick of unsalted butter + more for dish

How it's made:

- Ensure oven is preheated to 350 degrees. Butter a 1 ½ quart dish meant for baking.
- In a large vessel that is bowl shaped, toss together 4 tablespoons butter, flour, lemon juice/zest, ¼ teaspoon nutmeg, ½ teaspoon cinnamon, sugar, blackberries, and apples until everything is coated.
- Combine cones, brown sugar, remaining cinnamon, ¼ teaspoon nutmeg, almonds, salt and remaining butter in another bowl.

- Pour half of apple-berry mixture into prepared dish. Then top mixture with half of the cone mixture. Put remaining apple-berry mixture over top and top with rest of cone mixture.
- Bake 40-45 min. until apples are soft and top is golden brown in color.
- Transfer dish to a rack made of wire and let sit for 10 min. before consuming.
- Serve with ice cream or whipped cream. Yum!

Chewy Gluten Free Chocolate Chip Cookies

Preparation time: 25 min.
Complete time: 1 hour and 39 min.

Calories 119 – Carbs 14g – Sodium 249mg – Fat 7g

What's in it:

- 12 ounces of semisweet chocolate chips
- 1 ½ tsp. vanilla extract
- 1 egg yolk
- 1 whole egg
- 1 ¼ C. packed light brown sugar
- ¼ C. sugar
- 1 tsp. baking soda
- 1 tsp. salt
- 1 tsp. xanthan gum
- 2 tbsp. tapioca flour
- ¼ C. cornstarch
- 2 C. brown rice flour
- 8 oz. unsalted butter

How it's made:

- In a saucepan over low warmth, allow time for the butter to melt. Once liquefied, pour into a stand mixer bowl.
- Sift rice flour, cornstarch, tapioca flour, xanthan gum, salt and baking soda together. Set to the side.
- Add both sugars to stand mixer with liquefied butter. Mix with paddle attachment on intermediate speed for a

minute. Pour in the whole egg, egg yolk, vanilla extract and milk, mixing well until thoroughly combined.

- Gradually incorporate flour mixture until mixed well. Then pour in chocolate chips and mix until combined.
- Frost dough in the fridge for at least 1 hour.
- Ensure oven is preheated to 375 degrees. Form your dough into balls that equal about two ounces and put onto a baking sheet prepared with parchment paper. Six cookies should fit on each of your sheets.
- Bake fourteen min., turning pans around after seven min. of bake time.
- Take away from the oven and let cool on a rack made of wire. Indulge!

Jam-and-Oat Squares

Preparation time: 10 min.

Complete time: 25 min.

Calories 210 – Carbs 32g – Sodium 74mg – Fat 4g

What's in it:

- 1 Frosted pie crust
- ¾ C. strawberry jam
- ¾ C. oats
- ¾ C. flour
- 6 tbsp. melted butter
- 1/3 C. packed brown sugar
- ¼ C. granulated sugar
- Pinch of salt

How it's made:

- Ensure oven is preheated to 450 degrees.
- On a baking sheet prepared with parchment paper, unroll pie crust.
- Spread crust with strawberry jam, ensuring that you leave at least a ½" border.
- Mix oat and flour together in a bowl and add melted butter, brown sugar, granulated sugar, and salt. Combine well.
- Squeeze sugar mixture into clumps over jam.
- Bake for 15 min.
- Allow time for them to cool before cutting into desired squares.

Conclusion

Thank you for making it through to the end of *Blood Pressure Solution*.

I hope that the contents of this book were able to bring to light a health issue that plagues many individuals and how you can easily correct it and create a healthier you through the means of what you consume!

I hope that this book was informative and able to adequately provide you with all the tools that are necessary to achieve your goals of lowering your blood pressure and reducing hypertension before your next doctor's appointment!

The next step is to get crack-a-lackin'! Pick out which of the delicious recipes you want to try out first and make a grocery list! You will not know the amazing effects that these recipes will have on your life if you never get the initiative to try them out! I assure you, your taste buds will not be disappointed! It is not about sacrificing taste and satisfaction, but using correct ingredient combinations of food in order to help your body minimize the things that lead to heightened blood pressure levels and hypertension within the body.

Good luck my friends! You have made the great decision to embark on a journey that will eventually lead to a healthier you! Over time you will see and feel the difference these recipes will make. And your doctor will too!

Thank you!

Before you go, I just wanted to say thank you for purchasing my book.

You could have picked from dozens of other books on the same topic but you took a chance and chose this one.

So, a HUGE thanks to you for getting this book and for reading all the way to the end.

Now I wanted to ask you for a small favor. **Could you please take just a few minutes to leave a review for this book on Amazon?**

This feedback will help me continue to write the type of books that will help you get the results you want. So if you enjoyed it, please let me know! (-:

Made in the USA
Coppell, TX
09 May 2020